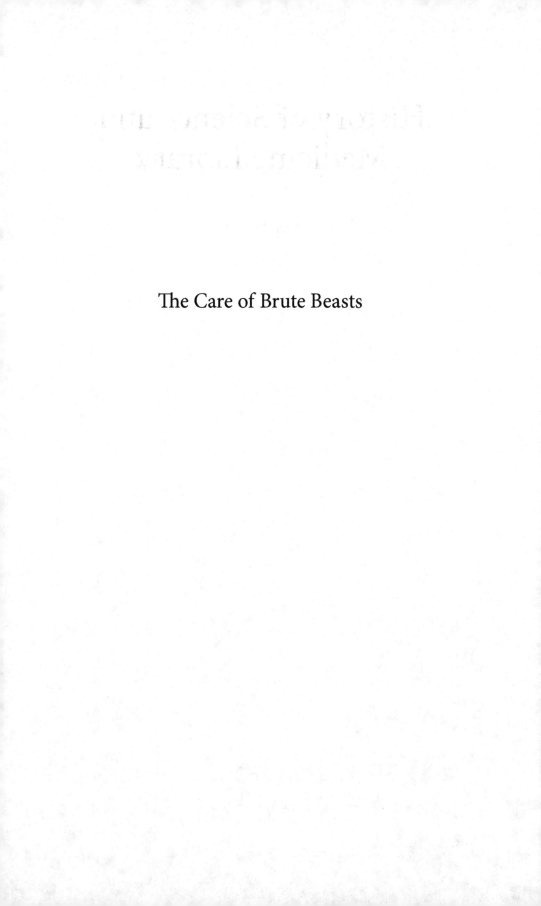

The Care of Brute Beasts

History of Science and Medicine Library

VOLUME 14

The Care of Brute Beasts

A Social and Cultural Study of Veterinary Medicine in Early Modern England

By

Louise Hill Curth

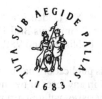

BRILL

LEIDEN • BOSTON
2010

On the cover: Detail of the cover of L. Mascal, *The Government of Cattle* (London, 1662). Courtesy of the Wellcome Library, London.

This book is printed on acid-free paper.

Library of Congress Cataloging-in-Publication Data

Curth, Louise Hill.
  The care of brute beasts : a social and cultural study of veterinary medicine in early modern England / by Louise Hill Curth.
    p. -- (History of science and medicine library, ISSN 1872-0684 ; v. 14)
  Includes bibliographical references and index.
  ISBN 978-90-04-17995-0 (hardback : alk. paper)
  1. Veterinary medicine--England--History. I. Title. II. Series: History of science and medicine library, v. 14. 1872–0684 ;
  [DNLM: 1. Veterinary Medicine--history--England. 2. History, 17th Century--England. 3. History, 18th Century--England. 4. History, Early Modern 1451–1600--England. SF 657 C979c 2010]

  SF657.C87 2010
  636.089'0942--dc22

  2009040279

ISSN 1872-0684
ISBN 978 90 04 17995 0

To my mother Joyce Ruth Hill and my favourite animals Vladimir and
Brigadoon (past) and Bessie and Pooh-bah (present)

CONTENTS

ACKNOWLEDGEMENTS

My interest in the history of veterinary medicine is due, in no small part, to the very important role that several dogs have played and continue to play in my life. Without doubt, I am in total agreement with John Caius' view in *Of Englishe Dogges* (1576) that 'there is not any creature without reason, more loving to his Master, nor more serviceable then is a dog'. That said, I admit to a general weakness for most types of 'four footed beastes' all of whom contribute so much to our lives.

In addition, I would like to publicly thank some of the 'human creatures' who have played an important role in the evolution of this book. These include Professor Peter Edwards, the uncontested expert on early modern horses, for his unfailing enthusiasm and support of my work. It is also a pleasure to express my gratitude to Professor Alan Booth for his ideas, practical help and encouragement through the many stages this book has gone through. Many thanks are due to Boris van Gool, my editor, and his colleagues at Brill. Finally, I owe a very special debt of gratitude to Rachael Cross and the Wellcome Trust Library, who have kindly allowed me to reproduce a selection of images from their outstanding collection of early modern veterinary texts.

All errors of fact or interpretation which remain are, of course, my own.

LIST OF ILLUSTRATIONS

INTRODUCTION

> It is a sad fact that historians of human medicine and historians of veterinary medicine seem to have relatively little contact with each other. Indeed, in the academic world, it is automatically assumed that a 'historian of medicine' is a person who works on the history of human medicine…One unhappy aspect of this is an appalling dearth of significant writings on the history of British veterinary medicine.[1]

This book is about medical beliefs and practices for animals in early modern England. Although there are numerous texts on the subject of human health, this is the first to focus exclusively on animals during this period. The main reason for this is probably linked to the dichotomy of medical historians that Roy Porter referred to over fifteen years ago. Today, the majority tend to focus on the experience of health and illness for humans over the centuries. These historians have been joined over the past decade by a small, but growing number of academics interested in veterinary medicine. Unfortunately, their writings tend to link the beginning of 'modern' animal medicine with the foundation of the London Veterinary College in 1791.[2] As a result, what might be called the 'pre-veterinary' period is either excluded, or fallaciously described as a time of 'unscientific' treatments administered by ignorant, one-dimensional and dangerous quacks.[3]

Such stereotypical conclusions about the history of early modern veterinary medicine seem to be based on two interconnected problems.

---

[1] R. Porter, 'Man, Animals and Medicine at the Time of the Founding of the Royal Veterinary College' in A.R. Mitchell (ed.), *History of the Healing Professions*, 3 (London, 1993), p.19.

[2] E. Cotchin, *The Royal Veterinary College: A Bicentary History* (Buckingham, 1990), p. 13; R. Dunlop and D. Williams, *Veterinary History* (London, 1996); D. Karasszon, *A Concise History of Veterinary Medicine*, trans. E. Farkas (Budapest, 1988); I. Pattison, *The British Veterinary Profession 1791-1948* (London, 1984); L. Pugh, *From Farriery to Veterinary Medicine 1785-1795* (Cambridge, 1962); F.J. Smithcors, *Evolution of the Veterinary Art: A Narrative Account to 1850* (London, 1958); J. Swabe, *The Burden of Beasts: A Historical Sociological Study of Changing Human-Animal Relations and the Rise of the Veterinary Regime* (Amsterdam, 1997) and L. Wilkinson, *Animals and Disease: An Introduction to the History of Comparative Medicine* (Cambridge, 1992).

[3] R. Dunlop and D. Williams, *Veterinary History*, p. 266; D. Karasszon, *Concise History*, p. 270; and I. Pattison, *Veterinary*, p. 2.

The first suggests that there was a medical void, or absence of a systematic method of preventative and remedial medicine. This is a surprising and even nonsensical idea given the major role that animals played in early societies. Their sheer economic importance demanded the presence of an organised medical system to ensure that they would remain productive members of society. After all, as Charles Schwabe has aptly argued, the main reason veterinary medicine was created was to keep animals healthy so that they could continue to provide benefits to mankind. This is not to negate the many moral and ethical reasons behind helping sick animals, but it seems likely that, out of necessity, economic concerns remained at the forefront, demanding that everything possible be done to protect their health.[4] As this book will show, this involved the creation of a whole social structure to define health and illness, in addition to providing a range of preventative and remedial treatments which were discussed in widely available manuals which targeted different types of readers.

A second reason for the stereotypes about animal health care is related to both historical and modern anthropocentrism. The underlying theory rests on the assumption the most important creatures on earth are human. This would support the view that human health was of both the greatest interest and worth to study. In the early part of the twentieth century this was illustrated in the emphasis of 'medical discoveries and elite [university educated male] practitioners'.[5] In 1951 Henry Sigerist defined those who studied medical history as 'physician[s], trained in the research method of history'.[6] Not surprisingly, the work of such 'historians' also displayed a tendency to transpose twentieth century concepts and beliefs onto the past. This included the negation of earlier ideas and practices which were 'inferior' to modern ones.[7] This is a problematic comment which suggests,

---

[4] C.W. Schwabe, *Veterinary Medicine and Human Health* (Baltimore, 1984), p. 2. For more on attitudes to animals see: K. Thomas, *Man and the Natural World: Changing Attitudes in England 1500–1800* (London, 1983) and E. Fudge, *Perceiving animals: humans and beasts in early modern Culture* (Basingstoke, 2000).

[5] A. Wear, 'Religious Beliefs and Medicine in Early Modern England' in H. Marland and M. Pelling (eds.) *The Task of Healing: Medicine, Religion and Gender in England and the Netherlands 1450-1800* (Rotterdam, 1996), p. 145 and M. Pelling, 'Trade or Profession? Medical Practice in Early Modern England' in *The Common Lot: Sickness, Medical Occupations and the Urban Poor in Early Modern England* (London, 1998), p. 232.

[6] H. Sigerist, *A History of Medicine*, I (Oxford, 1951), p. 31.

[7] K. Dewhurst, *Willis's Oxford Casebook* (Oxford, 1981), p. vii.

firstly, that early modern patients and practitioners were naïve and perhaps even ignorant and secondly, that only 'scientific' medicine is 'good' or 'right'. Such judgmental ideas not only deny the validity or worth of earlier belief systems of health and illness, but the way in which people chose to deal with them. Fortunately, most modern historians of human medicine have long since abandoned such ideas in favour of an exploration of more socio-cultural dimensions.

Veterinary writers, however, often appear to be stuck in this earlier form of academic thinking. According to Philip Teigen, the most common reasons for writing works on veterinary history are either:

1. To celebrate achievements and innovations of important veterinarians or institutions.
2. To explain who, what, why, when, where and how a specific event occurred.
3. To advise or recommend a course of action based on lessons learned form the past.[8]

Unfortunately, most are still very judgemental and contain at least some commonplaces on animals' healers being ignorant, shallow or even dangerous before the advent of 'professional' veterinary training.[9] The title From Farriery to Veterinary Medicine 1785–1795, for example, suggests that the foundation of the London Veterinary College in 1791 was a cataclysmic event which meant that it was no longer true that 'the most fortunate sick animals ... were those left untreated'. According to Leslie Pugh, this was because the majority of animal practitioners were 'mainly incredibly ignorant'.[10] Such dramatic language was toned down in the early 1980's, although many of the sentiments remain much the same. Lise Wilkinson, who wrote a number of works on veterinary history, continued to tell readers that until the 1790's 'veterinary medicine

---

[8] P. M. Teigen, 'Reading and Writing Veterinary History', Veterinary Heritage, 24, no.,1 (May 2001), 3–8

[9] R. Porter, 'Civilisation and Disease: Medical Ideology in the Enlightenment' in J. Black and J. Gregory (eds.) Culture, Politics and Society in Britain 1660–1800 (Manchester, 1991), p. 155; J. Swabe, The Burden of Beasts; R. Dunlop and D. William, Veterinary Medicine; L. Wilkison, Animals and Disease and C.W. Schwabe Veterinary Medicine and Human Health; I. Pattison, The British Veterinary Profession; L. Prince, The Farrier and His Craft: The History of the Worshipful Company of Farriers (London, 1980); L.P. Pugh, From Farriery to Veterinary and F.J. Smithcors, Evolution of the Veterinary Art.

[10] L.P. Pugh, From Farriery to Veterinary, p. 44; F.J. Smithcors, Evolution of the Veterinary Art, p. 247 and I. Pattison, The British Veterinary Profession, p. 2.

as such was non-existent both in theory and practice apart from a few treatises of diseases of the horse'. Despite the wide range of popular veterinary texts purporting to be written for animal healers, Wilkinson continued to insist that the majority were 'for the most part illiterate'.[11]

This theme has continued into more recent books on veterinary medicine, none of which focus specifically on the early modern period. Joanna Swabe has commented on how the foundation of the college aimed to 'remove the medical treatment and care from these purportedly brutal and socially inferior empirics' in order to 'place it in those of trained and scientifically educated men'. In 1993 Roy Porter pointed out that the 'standard story' about animal health care before this point was one of 'ignorant and cruel' or even 'barbaric' practices. Even the most recent survey of veterinary history, which appeared in 1996, negates early modern practitioners as being 'crude empiricists'.[12]

Such ideas mirror the thoughts of early human historians, with the idea that only 'great doctors' and discoveries about human health were worthy of attention. In fact, this book will show that early modern veterinary medicine had a hierarchy of healers and was linked to the same principles and practices found in contemporary human medicine. Based on time honoured ancient Greek principles of health and illness, healers focused on a holistic system that emphasised the importance of a good health regimen to build a strong body and to keep the humours in as balanced a state as possible. As later chapters will show, the holistic model of Galenic medicine had reigned supreme for many centuries, continuing into the eighteenth century, forming the core of the curriculum at the London Veterinary College founded in 1791. This should not be surprising to modern readers, for as Andrew Wear has pointed out, the 'culture of medicine had long roots in time and changed slowly ....but was part of the lived present'.[13] Although Wear was referring to human medicine, my research has uncovered a similar continuity of beliefs and practices in animal health care throughout this period. Such findings further support the growing interest in comparative medicine which may well help to 'modernise' the general study of

[11] L. Wilkinson, Rinderpest and Mainstream Infectious Disease Concepts in the Eighteenth Century, Medical History (April 1984), 28(2), 129–250 and L. Wilkinson, *Animals and disease*, p. 10.

[12] J. Swabe, *The Burden of Beasts*, p. 76; R. Porter, 'Man, Animals and Medicine, 19–30 and R. Dunlop and D. Williams, *Veterinary Medicine*, p. 273.

[13] A. Wear, *Knowledge and Practice in English Medicine 1550–1680* (Cambridge, 2000), p. 3.

veterinary history, a need which was pointed out by Lord Soulsby, the first veterinarian to become President of the Royal Society of Medicine, argued a decade ago.[14]

There are many reasons why it is important to study veterinary history on its own, and in conjunction with human health. Both offer insights into a range of contemporary social and cultural patterns. On the broadest level this includes the work of a spectrum of men and women who choose to treat animals. The large number of texts which focused on health and illness has much to say about the relationship between the printed word and growing literacy. It also encompasses the history of education, occupations and the emergence of professions. The examination of medical beliefs and practices provides glimpses of the ways in which animals were perceived and valued by the societies in which they lived. Finally, it can provide a background and context for understanding how 'modern' veterinary medicine developed and perhaps even some clues as to why.

This book cannot, of course, cover all of these topics. Instead, it aims to touch upon a number of key areas as a starting point for further research and discussion. By virtue of being the first academic text to focus on early modern veterinary medicine, it also covers a somewhat amorphous era. There are many ways to define the 'early modern period', although the most frequently used parameters are probably from roughly 1500–1800. Since this book is, hopefully, going to be a catalyst for further studies on veterinary history, I have decided to cover the entire period. This decision has resulted in an inability to provide as in-depth analysis of the various topics as I would have liked. That said, it has allowed me to do what Mary Lindemann has referred to as the 'mainstreaming' of medical history. According to this definition, the historian 'lifts it out of the confining limits of a disciplinary channel and refloats it in broader historical currents'.[15] In the case of this book, this has allowed me to begin and end at points that hold a great deal of significance to the study of veterinary history. The starting date is linked to the infancy of mechanical printing, the printed word and the subsequent boom in medically orientated texts. These early years were followed by a continuing growth in the number of books addressing both human and animal health throughout the sixteenth

---

[14] E.J.L. Soulsby, *Royal Society of Medicine News*, 15 September 1998.
[15] M. Lindemann, *Medicine and Society in Early Modern Europe* (Cambridge, 1999), p. 1.

and seventeenth centuries, which form the major part of my work. The book closes by looking at the eighteenth century, which illustrates a marked continuity of beliefs and practices despite the claim that 'modern' veterinary medicine began with the advent of the London College in 1791.

The Chapters

This book has been divided into three main sections and an epilogue. In order to provide a context for later discussions, the first two chapters will 'set the scene' through an examination of the contemporary beliefs about animals and ideas about health and illness. The second section will focus on the medical options that were available for animals during this period. Contrary to historical commonplaces, this included a huge range of choices. These two chapters will look first at the range of 'professional' and lay-healers in the 'medical-marketplace' before moving on to the huge variety of readily available 'popular' veterinary literature. The third section will continue with an examination of the structures of practice and knowledge, divided into the components of preventative and remedial medicine. Finally, the book will conclude with an epilogue which will examine the question of whether the eighteenth century actually experienced the birth of 'modern' veterinary medicine.

It is generally agreed that the ways in which animals were viewed was based on 'theological, humanist, scientific and legal early modern writings [which] represent animals as being the antithesis of humans'.[16] Although Christian theology did lie at the heart of early modern sentiments, the first chapter will suggest that it was economic and commercial, rather than religious or ethical, sentiments that provided the most support for anthropocentrism. There were on-going debates on issues such as whether animals had souls, could feel emotions and pain or be used for scientific experimentation. However, I believe that in the mainly agrarian society of the time economic considerations took precedence. After all, animals were a vital source of labour, food and other by-products which demanded that humans did all they could to protect the health of their animals and treat them when they were ill.

---

[16] E. Fudge, *Perceiving Animals*, p. 4.

Chapter 2 will move on to an explanation of the ways in which health and illness were understood and treated in early modern England. Ideas about what constitutes a state of health or illness are social constructs, which can differ dramatically between groups of people, particularly over time. The ways in which we view these concepts, organize and train medical professionals and treat disease are both produced in and reflect the structural features of a particular society.[17] In modern Western Europe the major emphasis is biomedical, based on the idea of pathogens attacking the body which results in disease. During the early modern period the focus was a holistic one, centering on building a strong body and preserving a state of health. Humans were encouraged to follow what we would now call a 'healthy lifestyle' and to provide something similar for their animals based on the ancient principles developed by Hippocrates and Galen.[18]

The third chapter will introduce the concept of the 'medical marketplace' for animals. Although this is a term that has previously only been applied to humans, my research suggests that practitioners and options for animals should be viewed as an extension of the 'human' medical marketplace.[19] Far from being made up of illiterate, barbaric practitioners, this marketplace included highly trained members of the Company of Farriers. It will also discuss the many other types of animal healers in the marketplace, many of whom appeared to have at least a rudimentary literacy, as well as the large numbers of men and women who are probably best placed under the label of 'lay' healers.

Chapter 4 will focus on the variety of written information available to all types of healers, beginning with the advent of the printing press in the late 15th century. This is a particularly fruitful source of material for medical historians, but particularly for those interested in animal healthcare. Most modern medical historians study socio-cultural aspects such as 'the experience of illness' by using a range of manuscript and printed materials.[20] Unfortunately, while the health of animals is

---

[17] K. White, *An Introduction to the Sociology of Health and Illness* (London, 2007), p. 5.

[18] L. Hill Curth, 'History of Health and Illness' in J. Naidoo and J. Wills (ed) *Health Studies: an introduction*, 2nd edition (London, 2008), 47–72.

[19] L. Hill Curth, 'The Care of the Brute Beast: Animals and the Seventeenth-Century Medical Marketplace', *Social History of Medicine*, 15 (2002), pp. 375–392.

[20] See, for example, L. Kassell, *Medicine & Magic in Elizabethan London* (Oxford, 2005), p. 4; M. Pelling, *Conflicts in Early Modern London: Patronage, Physicians*

often referred to in correspondence, there is a distinct paucity of records kept by healers and, of course, a total lack of 'first-hand' accounts. There are, however, other ways to examine the social history of veterinary history, with the least utilized source being popular medical books.

These included a wide range of publications aimed at many different segments of the public, from the highly educated to the barely literate. Although modern medical historians employ a variety of source materials, until fairly recently, the use of popular medical literature has been relatively neglected. There are now a number of studies that look at a range of issues from readership to what texts can tell us about contemporary society.[21] The study of veterinary literature, however, has consisted mainly of the magisterial work of the early twentieth century antiquarian Sir Frederick Smith. Written over a number of years, this four volume set follows veterinary writers from the earliest known manuscripts through the nineteenth century. It was a phenomenal feat for Smith to locate and read so many works. Unfortunately, his personal bias against 'pre-modern' veterinary beliefs and practices is very clear in his writing. In common with both previous and later writers, Smith uses the founding of the veterinary college as a dividing point from earlier texts.[22] As this chapter will show, there is ample surviving proof of a systematic, holistic model of health for animals in contemporary texts written by a range of 'professional' and lay-healers which provide insights into contemporary medical beliefs and practices. In addition, they offer a range of indirect and direct evidence about the demand for such information. As Ian Maclean has aptly noted 'the decision to reprint an author was made by directly commercial

---

and Irregular Practitioners 1550–1640 (Oxford, 2003); A. Wear, 'Medical Practice in Late Seventeenth and Early Eighteenth Century England: Continuity and Union' in R. French and A. Wear (eds) The Medical Revolution of the Seventeenth Century (Cambridge, 1989), 294–320; H. Cook, The Decline of the Old Medical Regime in Stuart London (London, 1986), pp. 28–67; and C. Webster, The Great Instauration: Science, Medicine and Reform 1626–1700 (Oxford, 1979).

[21] See, for example, M. Hunter and A. Gregory, An Astrological Diary of the Seventeenth Century (Oxford, 1988); W.H. Sherman, John Dee: The politics of reading and writing in the English Renaissance (Amherst, 1995); P. Slack, 'Mirrors of Health and Treasures of Poor Men: The Uses of the Vernacular Medical Literature of Tudor England' in C. Webster (ed.) Health, Medicine and Mortality in the Sixteenth Century (Cambridge, 1979), pp. 237–74; W.H. Sherman, 'What Did Renaissance Readers Write in Their Books?' in J. Andersen and E. Sauer (eds.) Books and Readers in Early Modern England: Material Studies (Philadelphia, 2002), pp. 126–130.

[22] F. Smith, The Early History of Veterinary Literature and its British Development: Vol. I (London, 1919 and 1976), p. 123.

considerations'.[23] The vast number of editions of works by authors such as Gervase Markham clearly illustrates the great and on-going popularity of the material. Furthermore, the material found in contemporary popular texts contradicts stereotypes that veterinary medicine consisted solely of harsh, dangerous treatments administered by ignorant, one-dimensional quacks. They illustrate the continuing predominance of traditional, holistic Galenic beliefs and the practices linked to it while challenging the claims of major changes linked that to the foundation of the first English veterinary college in 1791.

After the discussion of medical options and information, the third section will move on to structures of practice and knowledge. Chapter 5 will begin by explaining the principles that lay behind preventative medicine. Unlike modern medicine which focuses on treating illness, the contemporary emphasis was on not getting sick in the first place. As one writer reminded readers, 'one of the most important Businesses of this Life [was] to preserve our selves in Health'. Humans were also expected to provide similar care to their animals by using 'means to prevent diseases before they come upon them'.[24] The recommended way to do this was to have a healthy daily regime based on the Galenic non-naturals of air, motion and rest, sleep and waking, diet, evacuation and retention and the passions. However, although the way in which these factors could be manipulated in terms of human health has been widely addressed, there are no comparable modern discussions of their relationship with animals. The most general advice on keeping animals healthy revolved around not over-working them, providing a warm, dry place to sleep and appropriate foodstuffs for the season. However, a great deal of in-depth information was available in a range of printed literature on diet, as well as on periodical, preventative purging to ensure an even humoural balance.

It seems highly unlikely that people in the early modern period believed that attempts to maintain a state of good health could always keep illness at bay, anymore than we do today. Chapter 6 will discuss the types of remedial medicine that were available for animals when efforts eventually failed, and disease struck. Most treatments aimed to purge the system of superfluous or unwanted humours through the various orifices of the body. Despite the modern misconception that

---

[23] I. Maclean, *Logic, Signs and Nature in the Renaissance* (Cambridge, 2002), p. 53.

[24] P. Physiologus, *The Good housewife made a Doctor* (London, n.d.), sig. A2v and L. Coelson, *An almanack* (London, 1680), sig. C6v.

phlebotomy was the most commonly used procedure; texts suggest that various concoctions of organic materials were most likely to be tried first. Although modern works tend to suggest that these would mirror human remedies, this was not always the case. 'Shared' diseases were often treated with different preparations with cheaper or more easily accessible ingredients being used for animals.

The final chapter will examine the state of veterinary medicine in the eighteenth century alongside the common claim that it marked the beginning of modern, 'scientific' practices. Although there are various explanations for this, they all culminate in the founding of the London Veterinary College in 1791. In terms of simple common sense, it seems highly unlikely that the beginning of any new institution could result in such a mercurial change in medical beliefs and practices. As this book will show, the long established system of veterinary care in England continued through the eighteenth century and was, in fact, the basis of teaching in the new college. This raises the question of why, if such methods were indeed 'ineffective' they were still being used on animals who were only of value when healthy? Furthermore, what kind of people would have allowed healers who were ignorant and possibly even dangerous to inflict even more pain and suffering on their charges? I would argue that the period before the founding of the first London Veterinary College more than deserves serious academic study, which will benefit both our understanding of both animal and human health illness in the past, as well as today.

PART ONE

SETTING THE SCENE

CHAPTER ONE

ANIMALS IN EARLY MODERN SOCIETY AND CULTURE

The way in which animals are viewed and valued in a society depends on a range of factors and has changed dramatically over the centuries. Historically, the differences between humans and animals tended to be based on very different criteria than we use today. Veterinarian and historian Susan Jones believes that there are three main criteria that have been used historically to define animals: our 'market or financial relation' to them; our cultural beliefs and the type of interactions we have with them in 'a particular time and place'.[1] In twenty-first century Britain our definition of animals is fairly broad and biologically defined which tends to blur the boundaries. As a result, many scholars feel that twenty-first century animals are seen in anthropomorphic terms, as 'different but nevertheless clearly defined shadows of ourselves'.[2]

One of the defining features of modern human-animal relationships is the huge popularity of pets, or in current terminology 'companion' animals. According to some academics, the former is somewhat demeaning to creatures who were domesticated to fulfill the 'human desire for companionship'.[3] This emotional interest is linked to the 'animal welfare' and 'rights' movements to protect them from abuse in laboratory experimentation. Some have argued, however, that while many people have 'emotionally invested' in specific dogs or cats, most are unable or unwilling to see 'the larger consequences' of our societies on the natural world.[4]

Of course, the ways in which humans perceive and treat animals has always had some type of effect on animals. In the early modern period, these were molded by prevailing anthropocentric ideas. According to

---

[1] J. Salisbury, *The Beast Within: Animals in the Middle Ages* (London, 1994), p. 2 and S.D. Jones, *Valuing Animals: Veterinarians and Their Patients in Modern America* (Baltimore, 2002), p. 2.

[2] A. Room, *The Naming of Animals: an appellative reference to domestic, work and show animals real and fictional* (London, 1993), p. 1.

[3] E.C. Hirschman, 'Consumers and Their Animal Companions', *The Journal of Consumer Research*, Vol. 20, No. 4 (Mar., 1994), pp. 616–632.

[4] V. Conley, 'Manly Values: Luc Ferry's Ethical Philosophy' in P. Atterton and M. Calcarco (ed) *Animal Philosophy Ethics and Identity* (London, 2004), pp. 157–164.

contemporary theological, humanist, scientific and legal writings animals were 'the antithesis of humans'. Furthermore, every animal was intended to serve some human purpose, if not practical, then moral or aesthetic.[5] These creatures belonged to humans and as a commodity were valuable in an economic sense to at least some degree. Common sense dictates that it would therefore be imperative to do everything possible to protect their 'investments'. It also negates the idea that veterinary medicine did not exist before the late eighteenth century and that before this time 'the most fortunate sick animals ... were those left untreated'.[6] After all, as Calvin Schwabe has pointed out, the main purpose of veterinary medicine was, and is, to ensure that the benefits domesticated animals are expected to provide for humans are 'assured and protected'.[7]

In return for this care, animals were expected to produce a range of benefits for their owners. This would have covered a very broad range of tasks, from contributing labour or transport to providing different types of consumable goods. During the period covered in this book, it might also involve going to war, taking part in sport or being experimented upon for scientific purposes. There were also animals which were kept for other virtues such as beauty and companionship or sport as well as a host of wild animals.

The focus of this book, as in veterinary medicine, is on domesticated animals. Technically, this includes all those creatures whose breeding is or can be controlled by humans. It is believed that dogs were the first to be domesticated, followed by other useful creatures such as cattle, horses and sheep.[8] There have been many attempts, since ancient times, to categorize the many different types of domesticated animals. As might be expected, these changed over time according to the society and culture in question. In the seventh century A.D. Isadore of Seville divided animals into three main groups, starting with 'cattle', followed by 'beasts' and ending with miscellaneous, small creatures such as fish or birds. The first two refer to what we would now call domestic or wild

---

[5] E. Fudge, *Perceiving Animals: Humans and Beasts in Early Modern Culture* (Macmillan, 2000), p. 4 and K. Thomas, *Man and the Natural Worlds: Changing Attitudes in England 1500–1800* (London, 1983), p. 19.

[6] I. Pattison, *The British Veterinary Profession 1791–1948* (London, 1984), p. 2.

[7] C.W. Schwabe, *Veterinary Medicine and Human Health* (Baltimore, 1984), p. 3.

[8] I.L. Mason, *Evolution of Domesticated Animals* (London, 1984), p. 2 and W.H. McNeill, *Plagues and Peoples* (London, 1976), p. 187.

animals.[9] By the early modern period different, fish and fowl had been redefined as belonging either to the natural or domesticated world. 'Wild' animals served several roles, the first being as sources of food. The second involved sport for certain segments of society.[10] It is, therefore, hardly surprising that the general welfare of wild animals does not appear to have been the topic of much interest. As one early eighteenth century writer noted, the people of England lived in a land 'where one great Blessing we enjoy is, the being fenced by Nature from every Kind of voracious Creature'.[11]

This chapter will begin by examining the different types of domesticated animals found in early modern England by dividing them in groups according to the type of human purpose they served. As many centuries of writers have found, this is a very difficult task. The first section will therefore look at how this has been done over the centuries through the question of 'what is an animal'. Since I believe that veterinary medicine existed to protect valuable property, it will be followed by two sections on the economic roles animals played. Part two will look at the animal, agriculture and commerce, followed by the animal body as a commodity both when alive and dead, including their relationship with scientific experimentation. Finally, the chapter will end with a discussion of 'non-working' pets or decorative animals, a trend that has had gained greatly in popularity over the centuries.

What is an Animal?

In the early twenty-first century, the Oxford Dictionary of English defines an 'animal' as any 'living organism which feeds on organic matter, typically having specialized sense organs and nervous system and able to respond rapidly to stimuli'.[12] As previously mentioned, this is very much of a biological explanation, which clearly includes humans. In classical times, although it was generally accepted that humans and

---

[9] Isadore of Seville, *Etymologias* (Madrid, 1933), p. 57.

[10] H. Ritvo, *The Animal Estate* (Cambridge, MA, 1987), p. 16.

[11] R. Bradley, *A survey of the ancient husbandry and gardening* (London, 1725), p. 368.

[12] 'animal *noun*' *The Oxford Dictionary of English*, (ed) C. Soanes and A. Stevenson. (Oxford University Press, 2005), *Oxford Reference Online*. Oxford University Press. Acc. 12 June 2008 <http://www.oxfordreference.com/views/ENTRY.html?subview=Main& entry=t140.e2693>.

animals were related biologically, there were thought to be two main ways in which they differed. Firstly, that only the former were capable of thought and knowledge. Secondly, that all non-human animals lacked a capacity for 'intellectual activity'.[13] The ability to think and reason was a vital one, with Aristotle describing an 'intellectual hierarchy' which he referred to as the 'Scala Naturae' or 'Ladder of Nature'. This began with humans at the peak and animals and plants at various levels below according to their reasoning abilities.[14] That said, there were some similarities between 'savage' humans and 'wild' animals, as well as those that were 'civilised' or domesticated. The former, in both groups, could be dangerous and therefore only fit for hunting or other sport. Domesticated animals, on the other hand, had many virtues ranging from being hardy and able to adapt to being social creatures. In addition, they were able to appreciate what humans could offer them, could breed easily and were easy to tend. The most important factor, however, was that they could provide humans with a range of benefits.[15]

Medieval Christian theology, with its emphasis on 'human ascendancy' repudiated the classical view that there were some close links between animals and humans. According to the Bible, God had 'made man in our image' and given him

> dominion over the fish of the sea, and over the fowl of the air, and over the cattle, and over all the earth, and over every creeping thing that creepeth upon the earth.[16]

Manuscript accounts of the natural world, known as a 'bestiary' or 'Book of Beasts' described different types of animals, according to the purposes for which they had been created. Many are said to be based on the sixth or seventh century *Physiologus* which attempted to 'redefine the natural world in Christian terms'. Such texts illustrated the ways in which creatures which had been 'carefully designed and distributed' so that humans could fulfill their roles on earth. They also reminded readers of the need to 'regardeth the life of his beast' and to

---

[13] R. Renehan, 'The Greek Anthropocentric View of Man', *Harvard Classical Philology*, 85 (1981), 239–59.

[14] J. Serpell, *In the Company of Animals: A study of human-animal relationships* (Cambridge, 1996), p. 151.

[15] H. Ritvo, *The Animal Estate* (Cambridge, MA, 1987), p. 16 and F. Galton, 'The First Steps Towards the Domestication of Animals', Transactions of the Ethnological Society of London, N.S. 3, 122–138, quoted in E.F. Torrey and R.H. Yolken *Beasts of the Earth: Animals, Humans and Disease* (London 2005), p. 35.

[16] *Genesis* 1:26.

further the safety one of another'. In order to do so, it was necessary to acquire 'the knowledge of beastes, along with the knowledge of all the other creatures'.[17] In the sixteenth century, these were defined as 'all thynge that hathe lyfe, and is sensible...[and known as] beaste[s]'.[18] Therefore, although one writer argued that 'the Property of Body is alike in human and brute Creatures'[19] it was mainly the differences rather than the similarities that help to delineate humans and animals.

Much of this information would have been transmitted through the daily intercourse of humans and animals that lived and worked so closely together. It could also be obtained through written sources. However, before the advent of mechanical printing relatively few people would have had access to such materials. The growing numbers of relatively cheap, easily accessible texts available in the sixteenth and seventeenth centuries offered readers detailed, systematic descriptions of various types of animals including those which were very rarely seen in England. The Swiss physician and naturalist Conrad Gesner (1516–1565), for example, published the first part of his multi-volume *History of Animals* in 1551, to describe animals and their health. In 1607 the work was translated into *The historie of the four-footed beaste* by Edward Topsell who promised that

> the knowledge of beasts is profitable to many arts, sciences, and occupations ... which may be better perceived, by the particular practise [sic] and application of him that is studious thereof, then by any other means.[20]

Keith Thomas has suggested that the most common way contemporaries defined animals was as edible or non-edible; wild or tame and useful or useless.[21] Books that dealt with the care and/ or health of animals, however, suggest a very different focus. The most common means of categorization was to concentrate exclusively on domesticated 'cattle'.

---

[17] *Proverbs 12:10*; R. Barber, *Bestiary* (Woodbridge, 1999), pp. 6–10; E.L. Fortin, 'The Bible Made Me Do It: Christianity, Science and the Environment', *The Review of Politics*, Vo. 57, No 2 (Spring 1995) 197–223 (p. 198); K. Thomas, *Man and the Natural*, pp. 18–19; E. Toppsell, *The Historie of Foure-Footed Beastes* (London, 1607), sig. A3v and R. Allestree, *A new almanack and prognostication* (London, 1618), sig. B1v.

[18] K. Malik, *Man, Beast and Zombie* (London, 2000), p. 3 and T. Elyot, *The dictionary of syr Thomas Eliot knight* (London, 1638), p. 7.

[19] H. Bracken, *Farriery improved: or, a compleat treatise upon the art of farriery* (London, 1737), p. 9.

[20] F. Smith, *The Early History of Veterinary Literature* (London, 1976), p. 141 and E. Toppsell, *The Historie of Foure-Footed Beastes* (London, 1607), sig B2r.

[21] K. Thomas, *Man and the Natural*, p. 53.

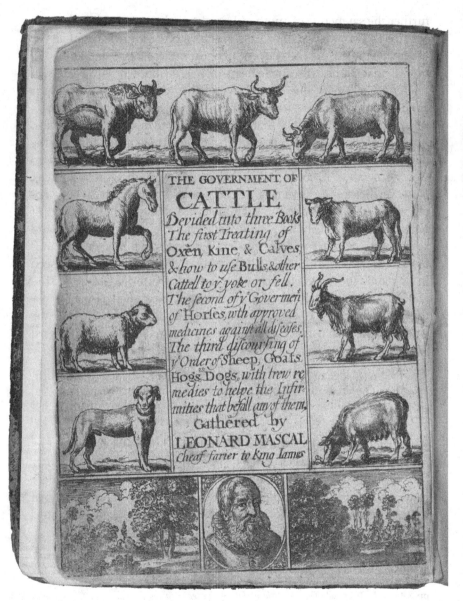

Fig. 1.1. Cover of L. Mascal, *The Government of Cattle* (London, 1662). Courtesy of the Wellcome Library, London.

'Cattle' was the generic name for working animals and is thought to have originated from the Latin 'capitale', (ie. capital in the sense of property). *The Government of Cattle* (see Fig. 1.1), first printed in 1587, discussed oxen, kine, calves, bulls, horses, sheep, goats, hogs and dogs.[22] Working dogs were also called cattle, with the exception of pets, such as lap dogs or singing birds.[23] They were generally further delineated into categories of 'greater' or 'lesser' cattle. The first type often included 'the horse, ox, cow, &c'. The latter referred to 'lesser sort of Beastes, as Sheepe, Swine, and Goates: and of Fowles, Geese, Peacocks, Duckes, Pigions, Hennes, Chickins and other poultrie', or deer, conies (rabbits) and other 'smaller creatures'.[24]

Although the format of T*he Historie of Foure-Footed Beastes* was alphabetical, Topsell actually divided working animals in terms of the purposes they served. These were basically broken down into those who produced 'marchandize' [sic] or by-products and those who laboured. The first covered 'cattell of all sorts' who were bred for 'fatting, feeding and felling' or those who produced 'butter and cheese'. It also included animals whose wool could be gathered while they were alive, or who provided leather and/or skin with 'their haire and wooll upon them for garments' once they were dead. There were also various types of 'cattell' who were valuable for their 'travile and plowing and carriage', as well as for riding for sport or in wartime.[25]

Animals in Agriculture, Commerce and Science

The kind of work, or economic contributions, made by an animal is clearly linked to the society and culture in which they live. Early modern England had a largely agrarian economic order, joined by a limited but growing commercial sector by the middle of the seventeenth century. It was agriculture, however, which was said to supply 'most of the country's wealth'. Furthermore, it 'moulded the social structure', as well as providing employment and income for humans.[26] This can be seen

---

[22] L. Mascal, *The Government of Cattle* (London, 1662), sig. A3r.

[23] I.L. Mason, *Evolution of Domesticated Animals* (London, 1984), p. 6 and W. Poole, *The Country Farrier* (London, 1652), sig. A1r.

[24] C.H., B.C., C.M., *The Perfect Husbandman* (London, 1657), pp. 211 and 293 and W. Lilly, *An almanack* (London, 1645), p. 27.

[25] E. Topsell, *Historie* sig. B2r.

[26] K. Wrightson, *Earthly Necessities: Economic Lives in Early Modern Britain 1450–1750* (London, 2002), pp. 110–111 and F. O'Gorman, *The Long Eighteenth Century: British Political & Social History 1688–1832* (London, 2005), p. 20.

in a number of ways, from how it influenced gender roles to how the yearly calendar of events was configured in both rural and urban areas. Their lives were 'regulated by the rhythms of nature', the weather and religious and secular festivals.[27]

Animals also played a major role in the running of an agrarian society, for as one writer noted:

> The Farm is of little use unless it be stocked with Beasts or other Animals that may be employed in the Labour and Work of it, and for the Supply of the Market and Kitchen.[28]

However, it should be remembered that not all parts of the country were suitable for keeping livestock. Instead, there were great regional variations in geography and soil which resulted in many different types of farming. Some areas in England were noted for sheep-farming and others for larger cattle. There were also parts which were more suitable for growing various types of crops. On the other hand, even farms that were mainly arable would have required animal labour. Heavy tasks, such as ploughing, had traditionally been done with oxen and bulls which were best 'fit for the draught' although 'cowes may be and are sometimes imployed in the same worke', although they were more suited for 'yeelding of Milke'.[29] Depending on nature of the land, the plough would be pulled by a team of up to eight oxen. By the late middle-ages horses were being used in some parts of the country to pull a plough, as they could work 1.5 times faster than oxen which would, in theory, reduce the labour requirement by a third. By the early seventeenth century, this resulted in a marked preference for using horses when finances and circumstances allowed, as illustrated in Figure 1.2.[30]

The socio-economic status of the owner also played in a role in the types of animals that would be owned. A farm that specialised in oxen or sheep would require at least fifty acres of good pasture to support enough stock to make even a bare living. However, regardless of what the farm actually did, a husbandman who owned more than just a few acres would probably have had several pigs, as well as poultry and

---

[27] M. Overton, *Agricultural Revolution in England: The transformation of the agrarian economy 1500–1850* (Cambridge, 1996), p. 37.

[28] J. Mortimer, *The whole art of husbandry; or, the way of managing and improving of land* (London, 1707), p. 148.

[29] G. Markham, *Markham's Methode, or Epitome* (London, 1633), p. 27.

[30] J. Brown, *The Horse in Husbandry* (London, 1991), p. 3; M. Overton, *Agricultural Revolution,* p. 80 and A. Hyland, *The Horse in the Middle Ages* (Stroud, 1999), p. 42.

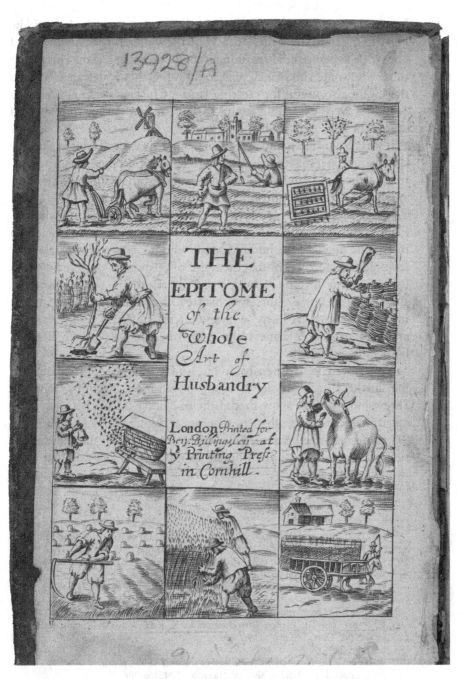

Fig. 1.2. Frontispiece of J. Blagrave, *The Epitomie of the Whole Art of Husbandry* (London, 1675). Courtesy of the Wellcome Library, London.

horses.[31] Even poor cottagers were likely to keep a pig which would be killed in the autumn for meat to last into the winter. Markham described 'the swine' as being 'the Husbandman's best Scavenger and the Husvwives most wholsome sink'. Since pigs could eat such a wide range of food they were also useful for clearing land.[32] Chickens were also easy to keep and were 'exceeding useful to the Farmer, Husbmandman and others' for their eggs, flesh and feathers.[33]

It was also usual to find at least one horse on a farm, which is hardly surprising given that they were seen to be 'the most necessary and useful Creatures to Man, in Peace and War; Enriching with their Labours, and pleasing in their Industry and Management'.[34] That said, there were a variety of different types of horses in early modern England who fulfilled a range of roles and tasks from hunting or carrying noblemen into battle down to the humble beasts who pulled carts or carriages.[35] It would therefore follow that the status of the horse would be linked to its' owner and the type of work it did. The most elite were known as a 'destrier, great horse, courser' or 'palfrey'. People falling in the 'middle income' bracket were likely to own 'rouncies, sumpters, hackneys, pads and hobbies'. Poorer farmers who only owned one or two were likely to have 'stots' or 'affers'.[36]

Horses were very expensive to buy and maintain, which made even the 'lowliest pack animal' a costly proposition. Records from the Shrewsbury Market show that of the 652 horse buyers between 1607 and 1628, 35 were gentlemen, esquires and knights, 94 husbandmen, 117 tradesmen and craftsmen and 406 yeomen.[37] Some urban dwellers, such as Samuel Pepys, hired horses in much the same way that a car would be rented today.[38]

---

[31] J. Thirsk, 'Agricultural prices, wages, farm profits and rents' in J. Thirsk (ed.), *The Agrarian History of England and Wales*, Vol II (Cambridge, 1985), pp. 117–18.

[32] G. Markham, *Cheape and Good Husbandry* (London, 1616), p.100 and M. Overton, *Agricultural Revolution*, pp 25 and 115.

[33] A.S., *The husbandman, Farmer, and Grasier's Compleat Instructor* (London, 1697), p. 138.

[34] A. Speed, *The gentleman's compleat jockey* (London, 1682), sig. A2r.

[35] K. Raber and T.J. Tucker, 'Introduction' in K. Raber and T.J. Tucker (eds) *The Culture of the Horse: Status, Discipline and Identity in the Early Modern World* (Basingstoke, 2005), p. 5.

[36] A. Hyland, *The Horse in the Middle Ages* (Stroud, 1999), p. xiii.

[37] M. Campbell, *The English Yeoman* (London, 1942), p. 206.

[38] See, for example, S. Pepys, *The Diary of Samuel Pepys*, (ed) R. Latham and W. Matthews, Volume 4 (London, 1971), p. 119.

Horses were also closely involved in the growth of 'consumerism'. Keith Thomas has suggested that there were three overlapping spheres of commercial activity in early modern England. These were small scale dealing between inhabitants of specific neighbourhoods or areas, rural-urban or inter-urban trading (food and other raw materials) and that between market towns and the surrounding areas (food, raw materials, manufactured goods and luxury items).[39] The emergence of a nation-wide carrier system resulted in the formation of new types of sales outlets, as well as the quantity of goods already offered in the long established system of markets and fairs.[40] Horses would have played a vital role in all of these areas, transporting raw supplies and finished products between the manufacturers, sellers and buyers.

Although main trunk roads to London existed before 1500, cross-country routes were less well developed. However, after 1600 the road system underwent a parallel series of modifications which helped to increase the volume of road transport.[41] By 1637 there were over 200 regional carrier services and by 1690 were over 300 wagons carrying both goods and passengers throughout the country.[42] While live animals could be walked to market, some of their by-products would have been transported overland. This included woollen cloth, which became the most profitable industry in terms of employment and turnover after agriculture.[43] England also had a strong leather industry which produced saddles, gloves and shoes. The majority of labour-intensive manufacturing was done in the houses of farmers and farm workers.[44]

---

[39] K. Wrightson, *Earthly Necessities*, pp. 93–98.

[40] D. Davis, *A History of Shopping* (London, 1966), p. 181; H.-C. and L. Mui, *Shops and Shopkeeping in Eighteenth-Century England* (London, 1989), p. 12 ; C.Y. Ferdinand, 'Selling it to the Provinces: News and Commerce Round Eighteenth-Century Salisbury' in J. Brewer and R. Porter (eds.) *Consumption*, (London, 1993), p. 394; L. Fontaine, *History of Peddlers in Europe* (Durham, N.C., 1996), pp. 186–8; M. Berg, 'New commodities, luxuries and their consumers in eighteenth-century England' in M. Berg and H. Clifford (eds) *Consumers and luxury: Consumer culture in Europe 1650–1850* (Manchester, 1999), 63–87 and N. Cox, *The Complete Tradesman: A Study of Retailing 1550–1820* (Basingstoke, 2000), p. 3.

[41] B.A. Holderness, *Pre-Industrial England: Economy and Society from 1500 to 1750* (London, 1976), pp. 142–143.

[42] P. Glanville, 'The City of London' in P. Glanville (ed) *The Cambridge Cultural History*, Vol.4, 17th Century Britain (Cambridge, 1992).

[43] C. Wilson, *England's Apprenticeship 1603–1763* (London, 1984), pp. 67 and 71.

[44] B. Coward, *Social Change and Continuity in Early Modern England 1550–1750* (London, 1988), p. 58.

Many domesticated animals were kept either for their by-products or to be butchered. It was generally cows who produced milk for consumption, but other animals such as goats might also be used. On its own, liquid milk would have been expensive to distribute even in a semi-urban locality, so it seems likely that much of it was processed into butter and cheese. Such foods, however, were high in the value relative to their bulk and were therefore better able than grain to withstand the costs of overland carriage. Some by-products such as urine or excrement could be used for medicinal purposes, although they were unlikely to have been transported.[45]

There were a variety of animals whose flesh was considered fit for humans to eat, including 'venison', which was the generic term for meat from wild animals. With the exception of poultry, the majority of domesticated animals that were eaten also fulfilled other tasks before becoming too old to be productive. The two main medical considerations for humans to consider before actually consuming meat from animals were its humoural balance and age at death. In general, similar types of animals shared humoural qualities. Sheep were predominantly cold and moist, although they would become warmer and dryer as they aged. In medical terms, this meant that meat from a young lamb would need to be cooked for longer than mutton from an older animal. Pork was considered to be the 'most nutritive', although it was too moist and full of humours for 'such as live at ease or are any wayes unsound of body'.[46] 'Ox-beef' was considered to be the best 'meat under the Sun for an English man'. While oxen who had reached their 'full growth' could be eaten, the tastiest, healthiest meat was thought to come from 'young or growing' beasts.[47]

The time of year that an animal was consumed was also important. In the winter, the 'inward parts' of healthy people were 'very hotte' which strengthened their digestion. This meant that 'strong meats' such as Beef, Barren Does, Gelt [gelded] and spiced and baked meats' could be

---

[45] J. Thirsk, (ed.), *The Agrarian History of England and Wales:* Vol.II, (Cambridge, 1985). p. 108; J.A. Chartres, *Internal Trade in England 1500–1700* (London, 1972), p. 46 and J. Schroder, *Zoologia: or, the History of Animals as they are useful in Physick and Chirurgery* (London, 1659).

[46] K. Albala, *Food in Early Modern Europe* (London, 2003), pp. 64 and 219; D. LeClerc, *The History of Physick, or an Account of the Rise and Progress of the Art* (London, 1699) pp.195–196 and R. Burton, *Anatomy of Melancholy* (London, 1621), p. 87.

[47] T. Muffett, *Healths Improvement: or, Rules Comprizing and Discovering The Nature, Method, and Manner of Preparing all sorts of Food* (London, 1655), p. 59.

eaten in moderation by most people. In the warmer seasons, however, when 'blood begins to heat and wax rank' it was healthier to consume 'meats of light digestion'.[48] 'Cold' foods were suitable for hot weather because they helped to cool the body. On the other hand, if the body was already cold due to the weather, ingesting such foods could lower one's internal heat to dangerous levels.

Nutritional guidelines were not the only consideration when considering which animals to slaughter. These included religious or cultural taboos, which made animals such as horses unfit to eat. The aversion to horse-flesh is thought to date back to ancient Athens and Rome. Historically, horses were to be used for riding and as draught animals, but only eaten to stave off starvation if no other food was available. The religious prohibition made by Pope Gregory VII in the early middle ages presumably helped to lend support to an already accepted form of behaviour.[49]

While there might have been a stigma behind eating certain types of animals, the same did not hold true for those that were sacrificed in the name of science. The foundation of the Royal Society in 1660 marked the beginning of what would become a long-term rise in the use of animals for research and teaching purposes. This was not a new concept as pigs, monkeys and other creatures had been used as proxies for humans ever since antiquity. In the seventeenth century, however, animals began to be used for a wide range of tests, including toxology and vivisection.[50] In the twenty-first century the word 'vivisection' is used to refer to all kinds of testing on living creatures. However, the word which comes from the Latin 'vivus' (living) and sectio (cutting) originally referred to dissection of, or surgical intervention on, living animals for the purpose of research.[51]

The practice of vivisection was open to debate throughout the early modern period and, indeed, until the present day. In the middle of the

---

[48] W. Dade, *An almanack* (Cambridge, 1620), sig. B2r; J. Pool, *An Almanack and Prognostication* (London, 1656), sig. B2r and W. Heathcott, *Specuulum Anni (London,* 1665), sig. A7v.

[49] M. Toussaint-Samat, *History of Food*, (trans.) A. Bell (N.Y., 1992), p. 98 and K. Albala, *Food in Early Modern Europe* (London, 2003), p. 66.

[50] K. Arnold, R. Porter and L. Wilkinson, *Animal Doctor–birds and beasts in medical history: An Exhibition at the Wellcome Institute for the History of Medicine* (London, 1994), p. 5.

[51] A.-H. Maehle, and U. Tröhler, 'Animal Experimentation from Antiquity to the End of the Eighteenth Century: Attitudes and Arguments' in N.A. Rupke (ed.) *Vivisection in Historical Perspective* (London, 1990), 14–47.

seventeenth century the major focus was on the morality of the procedures. Often referred to as the 'father of modern philosophy', René
Descartes (1596–1650) set out to prove that brutes are mere 'material
mechanisms'. Supporters of his theory argued that since animals lacked
any form of thought or consciousness, there could be no harm in
experimenting on them.[52] By the end of the century the debates had
shifted to the alleged uselessness of such experiments and their failure
to procedure sufficient, ground-breaking results.[53] There was also a new
sense of obligation to animals, led by the English philosopher and theoretical jurist Jeremy Bentham (1748–1832). His *Introduction to the
Principles of Morals and Legislation* (1789) argued that killing animals
could only be justified if it meant a speedier and less painful death than
would get naturally, or as punishment for causing damage to animals.
According to Peter Singer, this changed the tone from an anthropocentric debate about whether or not they suffered pain to a theriocentric
one where animals were to be protected for their own sake.[54] However,
as Roy Porter aptly noted, it should be remained that an awareness and
involvement in such issues would have been limited to a very small
number of 'elite thinkers', rather than the general public.[55]

Animals for Sport or Companionship

Keith Thomas' use of the word 'aesthetic' for one of the purposes which
animals served could be taken in a number of ways. Technically, this
refers to a relationship with art and beauty. However, in his text, Thomas
expanded this to include the beauty of singing birds, the ability of dogs
to 'display affectionate attachment' and even the lobster being 'an object
of contemplation'.[56] This line of reasoning could be taken further to
include the use of animals for sporting or entertainment purposes.
These varied over time according to a range of social and cultural

---

[52] D. Wilson, 'Animal Ideas' *Proceedings of the American Philosophy Association*,
Vol 69, 2, (November 1995), 7–25.
[53] A.-H. Maehle, 'The Ethical Discourse on Animal Experimentation, 1650–1900' in
A. Wear, J. Geyer-Kordesch and R. French (eds.), *Doctors and Ethics: The Earlier
Historical Setting of Professional Ethics* (Amsterdam, 1993), 203–51. p. 210.
[54] D. Wilson, 'Animal Ideas', 7–25.
[55] R. Porter, *The Greatest Benefit to Mankind: A Medical History of Humanity from
Antiquity to the Present* (London, 1997), p. 229 and *Flesh in the Age of Reason* (London,
2003), pp. 53–60.
[56] K. Thomas, *Man and the Natural World*, pp. 19–20.

factors and were firmly linked to the social status of their owners. Members of the upper classes might have a 'wilde beaste parke' where they could enjoy watching fallow deer or hunt, shoot or 'course' game. The latter would include the use of horses and often dogs to participate in 'those howres which he shall bestow in the cheerefull reviving and stirring up of his spirits'.[57]

Some entertainment for the lower classes also used dogs in "baiting", along with cocks, bears and bulls.[58] Erica Fudge has suggested that 'entertainment' which consisted of baiting and torturing animals was 'the most explicit and spectacular site of anthropocentrism'.[59] However, it must be remembered that this was also a society which also condoned spectacles such as public executions. To many modern eyes, it is only a small step from watching the torture or death of a human to that of other animals in the name of science.

Pet-keeping, on the other hand, was very much of a 'mass-market' issue and widely practiced throughout the early modern period. According to some experts, keeping animals for companionship implies that they are either substitutes for people or 'some sort of pathological condition to respond in a nurturing or parental manner' to animals. Others, such as James Serpell, see the love of pets as a more positive light. He thinks that most pet owners are 'normal rational people who make use of animals to augment their existing social relationships and so enhance their own psychological and physical welfare'.[60] This view is certainly supported by the various illustrations and representations of humans with animals that have survived the centuries. The love that binds them together is particularly clear in a striking terracotta figure from South American which is thought to date from c. 1100–550 B.C and appropriately named 'Kneeling Woman Kissing a Dog'.[61]

---

[57] D. Underdown, 'Regional Cultures? Local Variations in Popular Culture in the Early Modern Period' in T. Harris (ed.) *Popular Culture in England, c.1500–1850* (London, 1995), pp. 28–48; G. Markham, *Country Contentment* (London, 1615), sig. A1r;H. Peacham, *The Complete Gentleman: The Truth of our Times, and The Art of Living in London* (London, 1622; reprint Ithaca, New York, 1962), pp. 138–9 and G. Markham, *Country Contentments* (London, 1615), p. B.

[58] G. M. Trevelyan, *England Under the Stuarts* (London, 1972), p.65 and E. Griffin, *England's Revelry: A History of Popular Sports and Pastimes 1660–1830* (Oxford, 2005), pp. 98–99.

[59] E. Fudge, *Perceiving Animals*, p. 19.

[60] J. Serpell, *In the Company of Animals*, p. 147.

[61] L.M.Wendt, *Dogs: A Historical Journey* (New York, 1996), p. 171 and D. Harwood, *Love for Animals and How it Developed in Great Britain* (New York, 1928), p. 23.

There is also ample evidence both in English illustrations and texts dating back to the middle ages. Pet dogs were apparently so popular with members of privileged religious orders that Episcopal authorities repeatedly tried to suppress the trend.[62] Small dogs were seen at every level of society in early modern England from the royal court down to the humblest household. The Stuarts were known to be great lovers of dogs, which appear in many of their portraits. These animals were clearly of both a monetary and an emotional value, illustrated by James II who sent Queen Anne a 2,000 pound legacy from his dog Jewel, who she had accidentally killed while out hunting.[63]

Pet dogs were also popular with the middle and lower strata of society. Samuel Pepys' diaries had a number of entries about the "pretty black dog", named Fancy that his wife's brother gave her.[64] The value of such animals can be seen in the types of rewards offered for missing dogs, which was often the same as for horses.[65] Mr Buckworth, who produced one of the best known proprietary medicines called 'Buckworth's Lozenges' offered a guinea for the return of his dog. In *The London Gazette* of January 11 to January 14, 1691, it was described as "a very little black and white Bolognia Bitch, the Nose turn'd up, a white flip down the Forehead, two holes in each Ear, and a white whisk Tail".[66]

Dogs were also valued by other, less affluent members of society. At the other end of the spectrum were the little dogs who were carried everywhere by whores, or strumpets without which they "would be neither Fair nor Sweet".[67] There were also many others of various social rank who were said to 'delight more in dogges ... than they doe in children'.[68]

There are also many examples of other types of animals being kept as pets. These included birds which would be kept in cages so humans could enjoy either their song, or imitations of their own voices. By the Tudor period there were numerous commercial bird-dealers which resulted in a large market in London for singing birds.[69] In 1660,

---

[62] D. Harwood, *Love for Animals and How it Developed in Great Britain* (New York, 1928), p. 23.

[63] E.C. Ash, *Dogs and Their History and Development* (London, 1927), Vol.II, p. 108.

[64] R.C. Latham and W. Matthews (eds.) *The Diary of Samuel Pepys* (London, 1970), Vol.I, p. 46.

[65] *The London Gazette*, Number 2728: January 4–January 7, 1691.

[66] *The London Gazette*, Number 2731: January 11–January 14, 1691.

[67] Anon., *The Character of a Town Misse* (London, 1671), p. 7.

[68] J. Caius, *Of English Dogges* (London, 1576), p. 21.

[69] K. Thomas, *Man and the Natural World*, p. 115.

Elizabeth Pepys was given 'a pair of fine Turtle-doves' and the following year purchased cages for 'Canary birds'.[70] The popularity of this breed is suggested by the three separate ads for canaries imported from Germany in one newspaper. Larks, which had long been kept as pets in England were also considered to be very desirable.[71]

Conclusion

This chapter has attempted to provide an overview of the work and lives that domesticated animals led in early modern England. In the broadest sense, the defining term for the period must be anthropocentricism. The idea that animals existed purely to serve the needs of man has been a popular belief through the history of Western Europe. Animals were firmly seen as having been placed on this earth for the benefit of humans. Depending on the creature, this might include providing labour, food or other by-products, entertainment, companionship or a body for scientific experimentation.

It has been argued that anthropocentricism has been replaced in modern England by anthropomorphism. Erica Fudge, however, believes that seeing the world and all the creatures in it in our own image is simply another form of anthropocentrism.[72] The philosopher W.H. Murdy raises an interesting point by suggesting that it is natural for humans to value ourselves more highly than other creatures in the same way that a spider would feel that spiders were the most important creatures in the world.[73] That said, the question of why humans claim such superiority is one that has led to much debate and discussion. According to many historians, the strongest support for Western European anthropocentrism came from the cultural dominance of Christian theology.

The concept that humans were the central figure and indeed the reason for the existence of the world was substantiated by numerous

---

[70] R Latham and W. Mathhews, eds. *The Diary of Samuel Pepys*, Vol. I, 1660 (London, 1970), p. 232; Vol. II, 1661, p. 23.

[71] *The London Gazette*, Number 2732, Thursday, January 14 to Monday January 18, 1691 and D. Loades, *The Tudor Court* (London, 1986), p. 105.

[72] A. Room, *The Naming of Animals: an appellative reference to domestic, work and show animals real and fictional* (London, 1993), p. 1 and E. Fudge, *Perceiving Animals*, p. 7.

[73] W.H. Murdy, Anthropocentrism: A Modern Version', Science, March, 1975, Vol 187, 1168–1172.

Biblical references to the fact that animals had been put on earth to satisfy the needs of humankind, whether for labour, food, or scientific experiments.[74] There were many different ways that animals contributed to the economy which depended on variables such as the type of creature they were, who they were owned by and what part of the country they lived in. Since England was primarily an agricultural society, most had at least some ties to the land. Oxen, and increasingly horses, were responsible for pulling ploughs and transporting goods from one place to another. Sheep contributed wool, which was at the heart of the medieval economy, and was used to make cloth in the early modern period. They also provided meat and other food-by products, as did pigs, cows, goats and poultry.

Although few would dispute the use of animals for work or food, this did not hold true in the case of subjecting animals to gratuitous abuse or pain. This included a range of blood sports, from the cock-throwing of the lower classes to the torture of wild animals by hunting dogs belonging to the upper classes. There was also debate about vivisection or dissecting living animals to learn about the workings of living creatures. This practice was many centuries old and linked to the cultural taboos on 'mutilating' humans, which many medics felt left them with no other option.[75] Historically, vivisection was also justified by the idea that animals were being sacrificed for the good of the humans they served. In the early modern period, however, there were many people who felt that this should not occur. This did not have to do with concern for the creature involved, but rather the fear of negative effects on the morality or spirituality of the person carrying out the operation.[76] Others, however, supported the Old Testament viewpoint that 'A righteous man regardeth the life of his beast.'[77] This was clearly also the sentiment of the early American colonists who passed 'The Body of Liberties .... of the Brute Creature' in 1641, which was the first modern law to protect animals. It included the ruling that 'no man shall exercise any Tirrany or Crueltie towards any brute creature which are normally kept for mans use' and argued that it was 'lawful to rest or refresh them [cattel] for a competent time, in any open place that is not Corne,

---

[74] A.H. Maehle, 'The Ethical Discourse and R. French (eds.) *Doctors and Ethics: The Earlier Historical Setting of Professional Ethics* (Amsterdam, 1993), p. 204.

[75] R. French, *Medicine before Science: The Business of Medicine from the Middle Ages to the Enlightenment* (Cambridge, 2003), p. 27.

[76] A. Maehle, 'Ethical Discourse', p. 235.

[77] *Proverbs 12:10.*

meadow, or inclosed for some particular use'.[78] Unfortunately, such legislation proved not to be forthcoming in England, even though public unease about vivisection had become fairly widespread by the end of the seventeenth century.[79]

It seems likely that many of the people who opposed vivisection were part of the growing numbers who kept animals for companionship. According to Keith Thomas 'all symptoms of obsessive pet-keeping were in evidence' by the beginning of the seventeenth century.[80] Dogs, which were the first domesticated animals, appear to have been the most popular pets, with sharing many aspects of daily living, including 'spaces', food, names and diseases' with humans.[81]

The unifying theme that linked these animals together, however, was that all required medical care from time to time. Despite the many roles they carried out, the anthropocentric mood of the time ensured that every one was seen as a valuable commodity. Therefore, it was imperative that humans did everything within their means to try to provide their charges with a healthy lifestyle, prevent illness and treat their diseases. The following chapter will examine the contemporary ideas about health and sickness in order to provide a context for later discussions of preventative and remedial veterinary medicine.

---

[78] R. Ryder, *Animal Revolution: Changing Attidudes towards Speciesism* (Oxford, 1989). pp. 53–4.
[79] K. Thomas, *Man and the Natural World*, pp. 153–4 and 166.
[80] Ibid, p. 117.
[81] M. Jenner, 'The Great Dog Massacre' in W. Naphy and P. Roberts (eds) *Fear in early modern society* (Manchester, 1997), pp. 44–61.

CHAPTER TWO

THE PRINCIPLES BEHIND HEALTH AND ILLNESS

> Friend (if I may call thee) who ever thou art, that readest this small
> Treatise, if thou do it only for pleasure, it may add some profit also: but
> much more if thou practise. For what more pleasure canst thou have in
> any earthly imployment, then to recover thy sickly beast to health by thy
> labour and industry?[1]

As Michael Harward pointed out over three hundred years ago, the
successful attempt to return a sickly animal to a state of health could
bring a range of economic and emotional rewards to owners. However,
it must be remembered that historical concepts of 'health' or 'illness'
may not necessarily be the same as they are today. There are a range of
social and cultural factors that, in combination with time period in
which they existed, play a huge role in shaping our ideas about what
constitutes a healthy or diseased state. This includes the ways in which
language is used to define these conditions, the theoretical models that
lay behind them and the various mechanisms developed to cope with
them.

There is a large body of contemporary literature about what human
'health' means in early twenty-first century Western Europe.[2] However,
the most commonly used definition is still that coined by the World
Health Organisation in 1946. This states that health is 'a state of complete
physical, mental or social well-being' and not merely the absence of disease or infirmity.[3] The most striking part of this statement is the suggestion that a 'complete' state of mental or social well-being could ever
actually exist. There are other components which are also problematic,
such as what 'well-being' means, particularly in the context of 'social'.
Finally, it does not seem to include animals, but focuses exclusively on the
overpowering importance of human life and the relative insignificance

---

[1] M. Harward, *The Herds-man's Mate: Or, a Guide for Herds-men* (Dublin, 1673),
p. 3.

[2] M. Bury, *Health and Illness* (Cambridge, 2005), Chapter 1.

[3] J. Busfield, *Health and Health Care in Modern Britain* (Oxford, 2000), p. 3 and
WHO, 'Preamble to the Constitution of the World Health Organization', *International
Health Conference* (New York, 19–22 June 1946).

of defining health and illness in other types of creatures. That said, a recent survey of modern veterinary texts suggests that the predominant definition of health for animals is also the absence of disease.[4]

The contemporary idea that 'health' is the opposite of being diseased is firmly linked to the medical model of 'biomedicine' which is predominant in Western Europe and the Americas. Since this is centred on the idea of external pathogens attacking the body, it follows that a body which has been invaded by 'disease entities', such as a virus or bacterium, would no longer be in a state of well-being. In order to treat what is 'a pathological process or deviation from a biological norm' the modern medical profession relies mainly on technological interventions.[5] Furthermore, our system attempts to generalise causes of disease, how they will affect living creatures and how they can be treated. In many ways, this has turned the 'art of healing' in what might be called 'merely repair work'.[6] Although there has recently been a growing interest in social and/or psychological factors, for most health professionals the emphasis is still on finding new drugs or treatments to eradicate the effects of the attacking pathogens.

This is very different from the leading health model of medieval and early modern Europe. Alternatively referred to as 'classical', 'Hippo-Galenic', 'Galenic' or simply as the 'humoral' theory, this was a holistic model of health. Unlike the twenty-first century view that disease can be viewed in isolation as a 'generic entity', humoralism rested on the idea that 'disease was an integral part of the self...[and] the world of God and nature'.[7] In other words, the emphasis was on the individual and their experiences rather than on some external 'attacker'. A state of health could be defined as when the four humours within the body were 'in their natural state, or while they balance one another in quality, quantity and mixture'.[8] Such a functionalistic description did not suggest that a 'perfect' state of 'well-being' was possible. It also acknowledged

---

[4] S. Gunnarsson, 'The conceptualisation of health and disease in veterinary medicine', *Acta Veterinaria Scandinavica*, 2006, 48:20, 1–6.

[5] K.M. Boyd 'Disease, illness, sickness, health, healing and wholeness: exploring some elusive concepts', *Journal of Medical Ethics* (2000) 26, 9–17 and S. Nettleton, *The Sociology of Health and Illness* (Cambridge, 1996), p. 3.

[6] S. Kang, 'Cultural assumptions of medical theory and practice' in M. Evans, P. Louhiala and R. Puustinen (eds) *Philosophy for Medicine: Applications in a clinical context* (Oxford, 2004), p. 81.

[7] J.C. Burnham, *What is Medical History?* (Cambridge, 2005), p. 139.

[8] D. LeClerc, *The History of Physick, or an Account of the Rise and Progress of the Art* (London, 1699) pp. 195–196.

that being healthy could mean different things as every living creature was thought to have their own, unique 'constitution' or 'complexion'. However, as one contemporary author noted, it could be said that a healthy working animal was one who had 'the Faculty of performing all the Actions proper'.[9]

This chapter will begin with an overview of the basic principles of early modern holistic medicine, in order to provide a context for later, more detailed sections on preventative and remedial medicine. It will be followed by a discussion of the Galenic principles of the four humours before moving on to discussing the relationship between the humoural and the 'astrall' components. Generally referred to in contemporary texts as 'astrological physick', this consisted of 'The Natures, Signs, Causes and Cures of all Diseases...as they depend upon the Positions and Aspects of the Planets and Stars'.[10] Together, these models helped to explain how a person or animal fell ill, how the disease could be diagnosed and treated and even the eventual outcome of the illness.

An Overview of the Early Modern Holistic Model of Medicine

> As Fire, Aire, Water and Earth produce and give Life and Nutriment to all living Creatures, so the Humors, viz Choler, Blood, Flegm and Melancholy, are the principal Agitators in the Bodies of all Creatures, and, as it were compose, or at least preserve them; Choler by reason of its heat, being alluded to Fire: Flegm, by reason of moisture and coldness, to Water; Blood, by reason of its heat and moisture, to Air; and Melancholy, through its cold and dryness, to Earth.[11]

The basic principles of early modern medicine rested on what Carole Rawcliffe has referred to as 'an all-embracing, and eminently coherent, explanation of the human body'.[12] Although Rawcliffe refers exclusively to human life, humouralism also provided a logical, easy to follow line of reasoning for the health of all living creatures. In general, this held that living bodies contained a varying mixture of the four main

---

[9] H. Bracken, *Farriery improved: or, a compleat treatise upon the art of farriery* (London, 1737), p. 3.

[10] R. Porter, *Disease, medicine and society in England 1550–1860* (London, 1987), p. 23.

[11] A.S. *The Gentleman's Compleat Jockey: with the Perfect Horseman and Experienc'd Farrier* (London, 1697), p. 71.

[12] C. Rawcliffe, *Medicine & Society in Later Medieval England* (London, 1999), p. 33.

humours. This meant that each individual would have a different combination which would help to define everything from their physical
appearance to their emotional state. Any excess of heat or cold would
result in an 'unnaturall affection and state of the bodie', or in modern
terminology, disease.[13]

This holistic, individualistic model is an ancient one, dating back at
least to Hippocrates (c. 450 to 370 B.C.) and the body of writing which
later became known as the Hippocratic Corpus. This consisted of over
sixty works believed to have been written by Hippocrates or members
of his circle, including titles such as *Airs, Waters and Places; Epidemics,
Aphorisms* and *Prognostic*. These texts introduced the close relationship
between the environment and the health of living creatures. They also
established the concept that each had a unique combination of humours
and that disease was caused by different types of imbalances of them.
Although the humors were always in flux, the aim was to keep them as
balanced as possible.[14] At the heart of humouralism was the idea that
the macrocosm (the universe), which contained the four basic elements
of earth, air, fire and water corresponded to the microcosm of the four
humours found in the bodies of living creatures, as illustrated in Chart
2.1.

There were two central physiological principles that lay behind
humouralism. Firstly, that all bodies contained a mixture of the four
basic fluids or humors of blood, phlegm, yellow bile or choler and black
bile or melancholy, which were based in different parts of the body.
According to Galen of Pergamum (A.D. 129–c. 200), 'choler' was placed

Chart 2.1. The humoural theory

Universe	Humours	Features	Characteristics
Earth	Black bile	Cold and dry	Melancholic
Air	Blood	Hot and wet	Sanguine
Fire	Choler/yellow bile	Hot and dry	Choleric
Water	Phlegm	Cold and wet	Phlegmatic

---

[13] Anon, *A Physical dictionary, or, An Interpretation of such crabbed words and terms
of arts, as are deriv'd from the Greek or Latin, and used in physick, anatomy, chirurgery,
and chymistry* (1657), p. 39 and P. Moore, *The hope of health* (London, 1565), p. 45.
[14] V. Nutton, *Ancient Medicine* (London, 2004), pp. 77–79 and M.J. Schiefsky,
Hippocrates on Ancient Medicine (Leiden, 2005), pp. 54–7.

within the 'gall', blood in the liver, phlegm in the lungs and melancholy in the spleen.[15] Since the combination varied between individuals, it was the predominant humour which shaped and defined their 'constitution' or 'complexion'. In addition, it would help to determine the types of diseases they would be most subject to, their character, emotional state and the types of food and drink that would be considered healthy for them. The basic balance was set at birth, although these tended to vary somewhat as one aged.[16]

While Galen used humoural terms to refer either to specific bodily substances, or diseases, by the middle-ages the predominant humour began to be used to describe an individual's constitution. This led to people being portrayed as 'sanguine' or 'melancholly', terms that are still used in twenty-first century Britain. On a broader level, these phrases could also be used to describe the characteristics of different types of animals. Horses, for example, were generally said to be choleric due to their 'strong Martial Nature', which imbued them with 'infinite, great courage and valour, taking an exceeding delight in the warres'.[17] However, it must be remembered that these were general, broad statements and that even animals were known to 'differ much to their Identical Qualities and particular Constitutions'.[18]

The most common way to determine the humoural constitution of an animal was through the ancient science of 'physiognomy'. This was based on the theory that physical features could be used to determine what might be called internal characteristics.[19] While the earliest writings on the topic, by Aristotle, focused on humans, the science later expanded to include 'beasts'. In the late sixteenth century Giovanni Battista della Porta produced *De Humana Physiognomonia LIbri IV* which classified animals according to the nature and colour of their fur, other general physical characteristics or behaviour. He suggested that small animals were 'hot-headed' because their blood circulated at a

---

[15] N. Culpeper, *Galens art of physick* (London, 1657), p. 6.

[16] A. Wear, *Knowledge & Practice in English Medicine, 1550–1680* (Cambridge, 2000), p. 37 and V. Nutton, 'Humoralism' in W.F. Bynum and R. Porter (eds) *Companion Encyclopaedia to the History of Medicine*, I (London, 1993), p. 281.

[17] G. Markham, *Markhams Methode or Epitome* (London, 1633), pp. 1–2.

[18] Galen, *Selected Works*, (trans.) P.N. Singer, (Oxford, 1972). p.xin; A.S. *The Gentleman's Compleat Jockey* (London, 1697), pp. 25–6 and T. Tryon, *The country-man's companion: or, A New Method of Ordering Horses & Sheep So as to preserve them both from diseases and casualties* (London, 1688), pp. 2–4.

[19] M. Kemp, 'Medicine in View: Art and Visual Representation' in I. Loudon (ed) *Western Medicine: An Illustrated History* (Oxford, 1997), pp. 14–15/1–22.

higher speed through their bodies. Larger beasts, on the other hand, would be cooler and calmer than their smaller brethren. Other factors were also taken into account, including the features and movements of the animal's head and body.[20]

According to 'the antient writers' the colour of an animal could be used to determine their humoural make-up, which would help to predict their characteristics and behaviour. A horse which was 'bright Sorrell' was 'hote, fiery and of little strength' and meant that choler was the predominant humour. On the other hand, a 'cowardly, faint and sloathfull' animal who was of a mousy brown colour clearly had a melancholy constitution.[21] A phlegmatic beast would have either 'milky white' or a 'very white' hide and would be 'slow, dull and heavy' or 'cowardly, faint and slothful'. This would determine the uses they could be put to, with phlegmatic horses only being suitable 'for Cart and plow [and] to labour in Mills'. Swine were considered to be both melancholic and cholerick, humours which were evident in their 'fierce, savage and unclean Nature'.[22]

The humoural balance and constitution of individual animals would help to determine which seasons would be most healthful for them, as well as the diseases that they would be most prone to. Springtime, for example, was linked to Leo and Aries, which meant that it was a hot and moist season. As a result, although the spring was said to be 'the most comfortable quarter in all the yeare', this was not true for those who shared similar humoural qualities. The nature of the season threatened to cause a 'surfeit' or imbalance in the humours of sanguine animals, such 'bright-bay or dark bay' horses.[23]

In general, animals would be healthiest in the seasons with properties that opposed their humoural constitutions. The 'aestival' or summer quarter, for example, began with the Sun entering Cancer, which signalled the coming of hot and dry weather. This was good for phlegmatic sheep, as 'the powerful heat of the Sun in this season dryes

---

[20] D. Karasszon, *A Concise History of Veterinary Medicine* (Budapest, 1988), pp. 240–1 and L. Hartley, *Physiognomy and the Meaning of Expression in Nineteenth-Century Culture* (Cambridge, 2001), p. 20.

[21] G. Markham, *Markham's Maister-pieece* (London, 1615), p. 12.

[22] R. Porter, *Blood and Guts: A Short History of Medicine* (London, 2003), p. 27; G. Markham, *Markham's Master-piece Revived* (London, 1681), p. 7; G.L. *The Gentleman's new jockey* (London, 1691), p. 27 and T. Tryon, *The Way to Health, Long Life and Happiness: Or, A Discourse of Temperance* (London, 1691), p. 66.

[23] R. Allestree, *An almanack* (London, 1614), sig. B2r and R. Almond, *The English Horsman and Complete Farrier* (London, 1637).

up the superfluous moisture that accustometh to discompose him'. Choleric horses, however, would be prone to a variety of hot diseases, including fevers and jaundice.[24]

On the other hand, 'harvest', or the autumn, was considered to be a 'second spring' and therefore almost as propitious a season, best suited to those of a 'sanguine complexion'. Those of a 'melancholy constitution' would be most subject to disease at that time.[25] Since it was generally considered to be 'a suitable time to take Physick in', the satirical *Poor Robin* almanac suggested that it be referred to as 'the Physicians Harvest', presumably referring to the vast amounts of fees they could hope to 'gather'.[26]

There are many similarities in the ways in which early modern texts discuss these relationships for man and beast. For example, a phlegmatic person was said to be prone to 'Coughs, Catarrhs, Cold Distillations, Rheumatisms and the like', symptoms which would also be found in a phlegmatic animal.[27] In terms of physical characteristics, men who were choleric were 'swarthy, redde haird, or of brownish colour … very meagre and thin, soon provkt to anger and soon appeasted'. A choleric horse, on the other hand, was likely to be 'coal black' from the heat produced by excessive choler and was most likely to fall ill with 'Pestilence, Fevers, Inflammation of the Liver and other hot Diseases'.[28]

In theory, the 'habit or body' (ie constitution or temperament) of all living creatures would alter to some extent during the course of their lifetime. Children, for example, who were warm and moist, would steadily grow colder and dryer as they aged. Gervase Markham divided the life of horses into comparable categories, beginning with the 'foal age' which lasted for six years, when it was followed by 'middle age' until twelve years and then into 'old Age … which is past eighteen'. Although Markham suggested that it was imperative to determine the age of the beast before beginning any type of medical treatment, he failed to point out what the physical signs of aging were. Presumably, this was because

---

[24] Swan, *An Ephemeris* (Cambridge,1670), sig. B4r and T. Trigge, *Calendarium Astrologicum* (London, 1676), sig. C2r and (1667), sig. C1r.

[25] M. Holden, *The Womans* [sic] *Almanack* (London, 1688), sig. A4r and J. Bowker, *A New Almanack* (London, 1679), sig. C4r.

[26] Poor Robin, *Poor Robin's Almanack* (London, 1682), sig. C4v.

[27] T. Tryon, *The country-man's companion*, pp. 34–5.

[28] G.L. *The Gentleman's new jockey: or, Farrier's approved guide* (London, 1691), p. 27 and T. Walkington, *The optick glasse of humors. Or The touchstone of a golden temperature, or the Philosophers stone to make a golden temper* (London, 1607), p. 511.

his target audience would already know what these were. It appears that the majority of writers on such matters felt that such knowledge was too basic to be included. One of the sole exceptions appears in a book published in an early eighteenth century text which advises readers that the age of a sheep could be determined by the number of their 'fore-teeth'.[29]

The relationship between health and the four humors was further refined by Galen who is credited with developing the idea of the 'naturals'. These were one three basic types of phenomenon whose mixture would define whether an individual was healthy or diseased. The first of 'Thynges naturall' included the four elements of earth, air, fire and water which manifested themselves as humours. There were six 'Thynges non-naturall' which had the power to alter one's humoral imbalance: 'ayre', 'meate and drinke', 'slepe and watch', 'mevying and rest', 'emptynesse and replettion' and 'affectations of the minde'. The final category that could influence health consisted of 'Contra-naturals', which literally meant against the naturals or 'thynges ageynst nature'. These included pathological conditions made up of 'syckenesse, cause of syckenesse and accidents whiche foloweth syckenesse'.[30]

Although little could be done to alter either the naturals or the contra-naturals, it was believed that the non-naturals could be manipulated in order to protect health. It was generally accepted that the most effective way to do this was by following a daily health regime based on 'a steddy and regular course of living, agreeable to the institutions and laws of nature'.[31] Interestingly, the basic rules which included guidelines on diet, exercise and sleep sound almost identical to the 'modern' recommendations on how to live healthily.

As Chapter 5 will illustrate, clear instructions were widely available in the popular press on how to have what we would now refer to as a 'healthy lifestyle'. Although domesticated animals clearly had little control factors over how long they would be required to work, how

---

[29] Anon., *A Physical Dictionary* (London, 1657), p. 551; P.G. Sotres, 'The Regimens of Health' in M.D. Gremek (ed) *Western Medical Thought from Antiquity to the Middle Ages* (Cambridge, Mass, 1998), 291–319; G. Markham, *Markham's Maister-piece* (London, 1703), p. 6 and R. Bradley, *A survey of the ancient husbandry and gardening* (London, 1725), p. 373.

[30] L. Garcia-Ballester, 'Changes in the Regimina sanitatis: the Role of the Jewish Physicians in S. Campbell, B. Hall and D. Klausner (eds) *Health, Disease and Healing in Medieval Culture* (Basingstoke, 1992), 119–131.

[31] E. Maynwaringe, *The method and means of enjoying health, vigour, and long life* (London, 1683), sig. A7v.

much sleep they were permitted and so on, the majority of the non-naturals could be manipulated by the humans overseeing their care. However, despite attempts to prevent illness, it was clearly impossible to preserve a state of health indefinitely. Chapter 6 will show the two main ways in which humans could help to redress the humoural imbalances in their sick animals. The first involved introducing substances that would be retained in the body, and the second that would 'force' or purge the offending substances from the body. Both methods, however, required that the healer have an understanding of the basic principles of astrological medicine.

'Astrall physick'

> No Man can reasonably deny, but that the whole Prognostick part of Physick is govern'd by Astrology; and those Physitians which follow Hippocrates and Galen, in making that their Principal refuge, do wisely and commendably.[32]

Although some modern historians have argued that it was not 'technically correct', by the time of the Renaissance writers had inextricably linked Galenic and astrological medicine. The combination of the two was could be used for 'expressing the state of the body, nature of the infirmity, and consequently the cause of the same'.[33] However, the relationship goes much further than that, playing a role in every phase from infection, through diagnosis, treatment and eventual outcome. In general, the message they gave was that the role that the relationship of astrology and medicine was one of the most important parts of the science of the stars.[34] The idea that the movements of the heavens had an effect on all stages of illness was already an extremely old concept by the early modern period.[35] Information about astrological physick had long been easily accessible first through the oral and/or manuscript cultures. It was the advent and the dramatic growth in popularity of the

---

[32] J. Gadbury, *Thesaurus Astrologiae* (London, 1674), sig. A4v–5r.

[33] V. Nutton, 'Galen in the Renaissance' in A. Wear (ed.) *Health and Healing in Early Modern England* (Aldershot, 1998), p. 245; C. O'Boyle, *Medieval Prognosis and Astrology: A Working edition of the Aggregationes de crisi et creticis diebus* (Cambridge, 1991), pp. 1–2 and R. Allestree, *An almanack* (London, 1640), sig. C5v.

[34] L. Hill Curth, *Almanacs, astrology and popular medicine, 1550–1700* (Manchester, 2007).

[35] L. Kassell, 'How to Read Simon Forman's Casebooks', *Social History of Medicine*, 12 (1999), p. 8.

mechanical printing press, however, that made the greatest impact of the accessibility of information on astrological physick.

In order to explain this relationship, it is necessary to begin with a more general discussion about astrology which has played an important, albeit changing, role in western society for over two millennia. Although there have always been critics of the 'astrological' or interpretative elements, the discipline has only fallen into general disrepute in fairly recent times. Some academics have attacked its role in the past by arguing that it 'dominated the minds of the vulgar and uneducated' in fairly recent times. Others, however, are even harsher and dismiss it as being a 'pseudoscience without any scientific evidence to support its existence' along with other types of 'supernatural', psychic or religious phenomena.[36]

It is a word, however, whose meaning has varied greatly over the course of its long history. In his classic work on early modern astrology, Patrick Curry defines it as 'any practice or belief that centred on interpreting the human or terrestrial meaning of the stars'.[37] While this is an accurate description of the way it was perceived in the late twentieth and indeed early twenty-first centuries, it does not adequately describe early modern beliefs. As more recent work by Roger French suggests, the division of astrology and astronomy is a product of post-Renaissance astronomers and post Enlightenment historians.[38] I would suggest that a more accurate description should include the way in which the movements of the planets and stars were observed, recorded and analysed.

In fact, for centuries astrology was regarded as a vital part of the science of the stars, with astronomy, or the 'theorick' part providing the 'Mathematical Demonstrations and Figures.... [of] various Motions, Places, Magnitudes, Distance, and Proportions one to another', while astrology or the 'practick' part, used this astronomical material to illustrate and interpret the meaning of the stars and planets.[39] Despite the ubiquitous critics, serious students of astronomy and astrology in

---

[36] P. Thagard, 'Why Astrology is a Pseudoscience', *The Philosophy of Science Association*, I (1978), pp. 233–4 and H. Bauer, *Science or Pseudoscience: Magnetic Healing, Psychic Phenomena and other Heterodoxies* (Champaign, 2001), p. 14.

[37] P. Curry, *Prophecy and Power: Astrology in Early Modern England* (Princeton, 1989), p. 10.

[38] R. French, 'Astrology in Medical Practice' in L. Garcia-Ballester, R. French, J. Arrizabalaga and A. Cunningham (eds) *Practical medicine from Salerno to the Black Death* (Cambridge, 1999), p. 33.

[39] R. Edlyn, *Observations Astrologicae or an Astrological Discourse* (London, 1659), p. 5 and J. Moxon, *A Tutor to Astronomy and Geometry* (London, 1674), p. 112.

medieval and early modern England believed that they formed two inseparable parts of a single discipline. God was thought to be the force behind the movements of the heavens, creating 'the Sunne and the Moone to be the two great lights ... one for the day and one for the night'.[40]

Whatever their own views on the subject, most modern historians now accept the necessity of examining astrology within the social and cultural context of the time in which they took place. Many, probably influenced by Keith Thomas' *Religion and the Decline of Magic*, acknowledge the idea that historically, the study of the effects of the heavenly bodies was an 'intellectually demanding' discipline with ancient roots and that astrological beliefs and practices played in every sphere of early modern society.[41] In fact, Michael McDonald has suggested the influence of this work has radically altered modern scholarship, with astrology now being examined 'from the perspective of our ancestors, rather than from the [modern] point of view'. Tamsyn Barton, on the other hand, argued in 1994 and in again in 2002 that there was still 'huge scope' for examining the ways in which astrological practices and beliefs influenced all aspects of life in earlier times.[42]

During the middle ages, celestial studies were further broken down into judicial astrology, which used the movements of the planets and stars to make predictions about future events and natural astrology which was based on the general effects of planetary influence on the weather, agriculture and health. In the strictest sense judicial astrology referred to the movements of the planets and their influence on individual decisions and actions which would eventually lead to a

---

[40] C. Dariot, *A briefe and most easie introduction to the astrologicall judgement of the starres* (London, 1598), sig. E1r.

[41] K. Thomas, *Religion and the Decline of Magic* (London, 1971); P. Curry, *Prophecy and Power* and H. Carey, *Courting Disaster at the English Court and University* (London, 1992).

[42] K. Thomas, *Religion*, pp. 335–6; M. MacDonald, 'The Career of Astrological Medicine in England', in O.P. Grell and A. Cunningham (eds) *Religio Medici: Medicine and Religion in Seventeenth-Century England* (London, 1996), pp. 62–90; H.M. Carey, *Courting Disaster*; L. Demaitre, 'The Art and Science of Prognostication in Early University Medicine', *Bulletin of the History of Medicine*, 77.4 (2003), 765–788; C. Scott Dixon, 'Popular Astrology and Lutheran Propaganda in Reformation Germany', *History*, 84 (1999), 403–18; pp. 408–409; A. Grafton, Starry Messengers: Recent Work in the History of Western Astrology, *Perspectives on Science*, Vol.8, no. 1 (2000), pp. 70–83; M. Robyns, Medieval Astrology and the Buke of the Sevyne Sagis', *Forum for Modern Language Studies*, 38, No 4 (October 2002), 420–434 and T. Barton, *Power and Knowledge: Astrology, Physiognomics, and Medicine under the Roman Empire* (Ann Arbor, 2002) p. 29.

predetermined result. Such views were thought to be both dangerous and inaccurate by the medieval church, partially because this involved what was seen as 'the occult influence' of the stars and planets. Furthermore, many religious leaders felt that judicial astrology promoted 'pagan superstition' and challenged the basic Christian precepts of human free will and moral autonomy with the result that many people would sin while others would feel that it impossible to improve their lives.[43]

Natural astrology, on the other hand, dealt with issues such as the weather, agriculture, husbandry and medicine. Atmospheric conditions had ramifications for both community health, and that of the individual with unseasonable conditions resulting in crop failure, economic failure and hunger. Poor weather conditions could also heighten the severity of existing illnesses or, even worse, be the harbinger of plague.[44] They could have also a major impact on the health of readers, as 'unseasonable' conditions were linked to a number of serious illnesses.

Although there were many texts that could provide readers with highly theoretical, technical information on the relationship between the planets and health, almanacs and most popular medical works focused on simply offering practical advice.[45] Mark Harrison has recently argued that 'the belief that the heavens influenced bodily health persisted, both in popular and even in learned medicine, until well into the 19th century'.[46] This is supported by the on-going discussion of astrological physick in contemporary early modern literature throughout the period which this book covers.

---

[43] A. Walsham, *Providence in Early Modern England* (Oxford, 1999), p. 23; L. Thorndike, *History of Magic and Experimental Science*, Vol. VII (New York, 1958), p. 90 and E. Grant, *Planets, Stars and Orbs: The Medieval Cosmos 1200–1687* (Cambridge, 1994), p. 569.

[44] P. Slack, *The Impact of Plague in Tudor and Stuart England* (London, 1985), pp. 26–7.

[45] A. Askham, *A Litell treatyse of Astronomy, very necessary for Physyke and Surgerye* (London, 1550); N. Culpeper, *Semeiotica Uranica, or an Astrological Judgment of Disease* (London, 1651); R. Saunders, *The Astrological Judgment and Practice of Physick* (London, 1677) and J. Blagrave, *Blagrave's Astrological Practice of Physick* (London, 1672), sig. B1r.

[46] P. Curry, *Prophecy and Power*, p. 23 and M. Harrison, 'From medical astrology to medical astronomy: sol-lunar and planetary theories of disease in British medicine, c. 1700–1850', *The British Journal for the History of Science*, 33 (2000), 25–48.

Natural Astrology

One of the most obvious ways in which astrology influenced health and illness was through the weather. In a society which was still primarily agricultural, the climactic conditions were of widespread interest. According to one early eighteenth century writer, Hippocrates himself had stated that in order to 'perfectly understand the Art of Physick', it was necessary to 'learn thoroughly the peculiar Constitution of every Season and the Disease that happens therin'.[47] Since there were likely to be annual variations in the state of the weather, unseasonable conditions could result in anything from crop failure and hunger to heightening the severity of existing illnesses or, even worse, be the harbinger of new and frightening plagues.[48]

The idea that seasonality affects health goes back to time immemorial. Explanations of why this occurs, however, have changed over time according to the society and culture in question. In twenty-first century Western Europe, the biomedical explanation for the change in 'disease manifestation' is 'evolving host susceptibility, periodicity in pathogen abundance and transmissibility linked to the ever changing environment'.[49] In early modern England, however, the explanation for differences depended on the relationship between the individual seasons and the specific signs of the zodiac which they were linked to. The number 'four' figured strongly in early modern astrology with a universe divided into the four basic elements of fire, water, earth and air. These characteristics were mirrored in the bodies of all living creatures, as well as in their life cycle which was also broken into four phases, beginning with a warm and moist youth and moving on to a cold and dry old age. Each of the four seasons of the year was similarly linked, with spring being hot and moist, summer hot and dry, autumn cold and dry, followed by winter which was cold and wet.

Each quarter would begin when the sun moved into a certain sign, such as winter starting when the sun moved into Capricorn. Since this was based on astrological calculations, the exact time when this would happen would vary each year. Almanacs provided the exact timings of

---

[47] Hippocrates, *The aphorisms of Hippocrates* (London, 1708), p. iv.

[48] J.D. Post, 'Climactic Variability and the European Morality Wave of the Early 1740's', *Journal of Interdisciplinary History*, XV (Summer, 1984), pp. 2–9 and P. Slack, *The Impact of Plague in Tudor and Stuart England* (London, 1985), pp. 26–7.

[49] E.N. Naumova, 'Mystery of Seasonality: Getting the Rhythm of Nature', *Journal of Public Health Policy* (2006), 27, 2–12.

such events along with predictions of the effects this would have on the weather, agriculture and health.[50] Most also included more detailed descriptions of how each season could affect the health of both man and beast. On the broadest level, this included lists of diseases that were common in each quarter or what times of the year were best for carrying out various medical procedures. Springtime, for example, was linked to Leo and Aries, which meant that it was a hot and moist season and therefore paralleled creatures with a predominantly sanguine complexion. As a result, although the spring was said to be 'the most comfortable quarter in all the yeare', this was 'comparatively such', as it could still cause humoral imbalances in someone with a similar constitution.[51]

'Foule weather', however, could appear at any time of year resulting in 'enduring harme to Cattel' either through 'lean crops' or 'putrefaction of the Fruites of the Earth'. An exceptionally hot spring of summer signified droughts, the failure of crops and the death of working animals. On the other extreme, a severely cold winter would contribute to 'malignancy amongst small Cattels', and excessively wet years would result in widespread sheep-rot.[52]

The movements of the planets were not the only factor in astrological physick. Unusual or rarely occurring configurations were thought to have a serious impact on living creatures. Although some astral events were thought to cause war or crop failure, others were specifically linked to health problems in both man and beast. The exact consequences varied, and sometimes were thought only to affect certain forms of 'cattel'.[53]

Conjunctions involving Saturn were particularly worrying, as the planet was 'the general significator of Labour Disturbance, Anxiety, Melancholy, Poverty, Treachery, Malice, Disgrace &c'. Almanacs, which were produced annually, provided numerous warnings about the effects such conjunctions would have on animals. William Lilly warned that a conjunction of Saturn in the fifth house could result in:

---

[50] W. Andrews, *News from the starres* (London, 1680), sig. C4v.

[51] R. Allestree, *A new almanacke and prognostication* (London, 1614), sig. B2r and W. Clarke, *A new almanacke* (London, 1668), sig. B4r.

[52] J. Woodhouse, *A new almanacke and prognostication* (London, 1619), sig. A4v; T. Hill, *A necessary almanack* (London, 1572), sig. B3r and R. Saunders, *Apollo Anglicanus* (London, 1674), sig. B1v.

[53] K. Thomas, *Religion*, p. 338 and H. Coley, *Nuncious Coelestis* (London, 1676), sig. C4r.

detriment, hinderance, losse, consumption, and destruction of four-footed beasts, both greater and smaller, and especially if those are most useful for man, as the Ox, the Horse, Cow, Asse, the Hog, Sheep, Deer, Conny, &c.[54]

James Baston explained that the conjunction of Saturn and Mars in Virgo would result in a sickly autumn for animals. The conjunction in the spring of 1673 was also predicted to be a time of 'sickness and death of oxen and great cattel', while the 'oppositions of the planets' in January 1682 forewarned of ill health in animals for the entire year.[55] Thirteen years later, Saturn was again due to affect the health of those who laboured for the reader, this time through a conjunction of Saturn and Mars in Capricorn. Almanacs warned that this would result in 'much Detriment and Damage to small Cattel, a Rot or Murrain ranging amongst them, even to the Destruction of whole flocks'.[56]

Eclipses and comets also threatened the health of animals. William Lilly cautioned his readers that a forthcoming eclipse meant that 'The Country-man will also be very sad upon the unusual misfortunes happening unto him, and unto his flocks of four footed beasts, especially Horses, Oxen and such like of the kinds of the greater Cattle, as also rot of sheep'.[57] In 1681, Thomas Fowle prophesised that, while the coming eclipse would destroy animals 'that are prejudicial to man-kind… all Creatures fit for the use of man do now increase'. Fourteen years later, Fowle warned that the impending eclipse would bring 'great losses and decay in their Estate, Cattels and Treasure; it portends death to the greater sort of Cattel, as the Ox, Cow, Horse, or such like'. Other types of animals, presumably, would have remained untouched.[58]

Meteors or comets brought trouble in their wake, with their shape often indicating both the type of coming misfortune and the kind of creatures it would affect. The former, made up of 'mineral and watery exhalations' were considered to be the 'manifestations of earthly

---

[54] W. Lilly, *Merlinus Anglicus Junior* (London, 1644), p. 12.

[55] J. Baston, *Mercurius hermeticus ephemeris* (London, 1657), sig. B5v; C. Atkinson, *Panterpre: or, a pleasant almanack* (London, 1673), sig. C2r and H. Coley, *Nuncious Coelestis* (London,1682), sig. C2v.

[56] J. Bucknall, *The Shepherds* [sic] almanack (London, 1675), sig. C4v, J. Tanner, *Angelus Britannicus* (London, 1697), sig. C3v and W. G. Bell, *The Great Plague in London in 1665* (London, 1924), p. 2.

[57] W. Lilly, *Merlinus*, 1644, p. 12.

[58] T. Fowle, *Speculum uranicum* (London, 1695), sig. B1r.

effluvia'.[59] The shape and size of meteors would determine what effects they would have on health. 'Many meteors of unequall shape', for example, foretold a period of 'infected ayre'. Comets were also linked to the onslaught of disease. A big comet in March 1665 was thought to have ushered in the great plague in London. Eight years later, a small comet resulted in 'great detriment and many infirmities to those Cattel most useful for man, as Horses, Oxen, Sheep and Hogs'.[60]

Although modern readers might view this advice with some scepticism, contemporary sources suggest that these warnings would have been taken extremely seriously. One excellent illustration can be found in John Evelyn's diary for March 1652 in which he refers to:

> That celebrated Eclipse of the Sun, so much threatened by the Astrologers, & had so exceedingly alarm'd the whole Nation, so as hardly any would worke, none stir out of their houses.[61]

In Oxford, a 'blazing star' was reported as being visible from December 1664 through to the latter end of January. Anthony Wood claimed that this had led to 'prodigious births …. [and] the devill let loose to possess people' as well as earthquakes and plague.[62] Samuel Pepys referred to the fear provoked by a meteor in May 1668. He further commented on the 'many clusters of people talking of it' and how

> The world doth make much discourse of it – their apprehensions being mighty full of the rest of the City to be burned, and the papists to cut their throats.[63]

Such warnings may have been seen differently by more pragmatic people. This advance notice would have given them time to try to do something about protecting their own health, and that of their animals. Leading a good, sin-free life was one of the ways in which this could, hopefully, be done. Although it was widely believed that animals were

---

[59] V. Jankovic, *Reading the skies: a cultural history of English weather, 1650–1820* (Manchester, 2000), p. 27.

[60] J. Manning, *A new booke, intituled, I am for you all, complexions castle* (London, 1604), sig. A8r; R. Saunders, 1667, sig. C3r; A. Geneva, *Astrology and the Seventeenth Century Mind: William Lilly and the Language of the Stars* (Manchester, 1995), p. 87; W.G. Bell, *The Great Plague*, p. 2; and W. Lilly, *Merlinus anglicanus junior* (London, 1643), sig. B2r.

[61] J. Evelyn, *The Diary of John Evelyn*, ed. G. de la Bedoyere (Woodbridge, Suffolk, 1995), p. 82.

[62] A. Wood, *Wood's Life and Times*, Vol. II, ed. A. Clark (Oxford, 1892), pp. 53–4.

[63] S. Pepys, *The Diary of Samuel Pepys*, Vol. IX, eds. R.C. Latham and W. Matthews (London, 1976), p. 208.

incapable of sinning, comparable behaviour in their owners could
result in their own sickness. The following chapter will discuss the different types of options people had for treating, or obtaining help, for
their sick animals.

Conclusion

Every society and culture has its own ways of defining what health and
illness mean and how they can be dealt with. The predominant model
in twenty-first century Western Europe is that of 'biomedicine', which
rests on the idea of pathogens attacking the body. This is an ontological
model which views disease as a real, independent entity which suggests
that it is the bacteria or virus that is being treated, not the individual.
These generic diseases 'cause' a pathological state which will produce
the same types of effects, and therefore can be treated in a similar way,
in all patients. Once the cause is identified, treatment can begin and, in
theory, lead to comparable outcomes.[64]

The medical system of early modern England was dramatically different, being based on a holistic, orthodox, traditional mixture of astrological and Galenic beliefs and practices. Their major emphasis was on
having a healthy lifestyle, in order to maintain or build a strong body
better able to fight out disease. Health was seen within a holistic framework which looked at the entire physical and social dimensions of each
individual. It was believed that there were multiple, interacting causes
behind disease. Since every individual had a unique constitution and
mix of humours, it meant that each could react in different ways to the
disorder, the course it would take and the eventual outcome.

As one contemporary writer noted, 'Physic without Astrology is like
a Cloud without Rain'.[65] Astrology and astronomy, which were two
parts of the same science, helped to explain the mechanism behind disease. Since God could use the heavens to communicate his will to all
living creatures, it followed that he could punish them through those
means. The movements of the stars and planets were believed to have
the power to cause imbalances within living creatures, resulting in illness and disease. These were orchestrated by God, who was the 'chief

---

[64] D.G. Bates, 'Why Not Call Modern Medicine Alternative'?, *Perspectives in Biology
and Medicine*, 43.4 (2000) 502–518.
[65] R. Saunders, *Apollo anglicanus* (London, 1681), sig. A6v.

Gouvernour' of the heavens, and who could choose to cause disease, plagues or epidemics to strike individual humans or animals, whole communities or even nations.[66] That said, God also provided a range of organic and inorganic ingredients to be used medicinally, as well as endowing some individuals with the ability to treat poorly humans and animals.

---

[66] A. Chapman, 'Astrological Medicine' in A. Wear (ed.) *Health, Medicine and Mortality in the Sixteenth Century* (Cambridge, 1979), p. 286.

PART TWO

STRUCTURES OF KNOWLEDGE

CHAPTER THREE

THE MEDICAL MARKETPLACE FOR ANIMALS

As previously discussed, the discipline of medical history has experienced many changes over the past few decades. In human medicine, the major focus is now on the ways in which people understood, diagnosed and treated physical or mental disorders. For most historians, these studies are placed within the framework of a 'medical marketplace' consisting of various healers, treatments and medical products. This model includes what were once referred to as the traditional tripartite division of physicians, surgeons and apothecaries, along with various types of quacks, clergymen, midwives, magical healers, herbalists, drug dealers and a host of other less categorical healers.[1] The unifying factor behind these practitioners was that they all focused on the health of humans. Such anthropocentric attitudes, therefore, ignore the comparable range of practitioners and medical options for animals which I feel should be included under the heading of the medical marketplace.[2]

As with many other terms, there is some debate over whether 'medical marketplace' adequately describes the myriad of choices available. Many historians have argued that this infers a purely commercial scenario staffed by 'qualified' practitioners.[3] According to English Common Law anyone could call themselves a healer, prescribe and administer

---

[1] H. Cook, *The Decline of the Old Medical Regime in Stuart London* (London, 1986), pp. 28–67; A. Wear, 'Medical Practice in Late Seventeenth and Early Eighteenth Century England: Continuity and Union' in R. French and A. Wear (eds) *The Medical Revolution of the Seventeenth Century* (Cambridge, 1989), 294–320, p. 302 and A. Wear, 'The Popularization of Medicine in Early Modern England' in R. Porter (ed.) *The Popularization of Medicine 1650–1850* (London, 1992), p. 17.

[2] L. Hill Curth, 'The Care of the Brute Beast: Animals and the Seventeenth-Century Medical Marketplace', *Social History of Medicine*, 15 (2002), pp. 375–392.

[3] A. Wear, 'Religious beliefs and medicine in early modern England' in Hilary Marland and Margaret Pelling (eds.) *The task of healing: Medicine, religion and gender in England and the Netherlands 1450-1800* (Rotterdam, 1996), 145–170, p. 145; H. Cook, *The Decline of the Old Medical Regime*, p. 28; R. Porter, 'The Peoples Health in Georgian England' in T. Harris (ed.), *Popular Culture in England c.1500–1850* (London, 1995), p. 125 and M. Pelling, 'Trade or Profession? Medical Practice in Early Modern England' in idem, *The Common Lot: Sickness, Medical Occupations and the Urban Poor in Early Modern England* (London, 1998), 230–58, p. 23.

medical treatment. This resulted in a large number of people who bartered services in return goods or other services, or even for free for
charitable or neighbourly reasons. These might include members of the
clergy or other charitable providers, as well as otherwise 'commercial'
practitioners who offered complementary consultations or free drugs.
For humans, the most frequent provider of medical assistance was
probably the housewife, who saw to the needs of her own household.
Andrew Wear has argued that the presence of such healers who either
bartered or offered their services for free makes 'exchange market'
a more accurate term than 'medical marketplace'.[4] On the other hand,
it could be said that so-called 'free' services actually had a cost attached
to them, and therefore were 'commercial' transactions. Clergymen may
have required a committement to being 'Godly' in return for their services. Others may have been adhering to accepted behavioural norms
and medical practitioners who provided free consultations hoped to
eventually acquiring a paying patient.

This chapter will discuss the range of men and women who provided similar care for animals. Although these options could form a
separate 'animal medical marketplace', they were not necessarily mutu-
ally exclusive and therefore I feel should be integrated into the current
model. As with human health care, there were a variety of commercial
and non-commercial medical providers for animals. This included a
hierarchy of healers similar to that found in human medicine, the
choice of whom might depend on the type of animal to be treated and
the resources of its owners. At the top were members of the Farriers
Company who had a legal monopoly to treat horses within the city and
a seven mile radius of London.[5] They were followed by various types of
practitioners such as self-styled farriers, 'leeches' or 'animal doctors'.
As with human health care, it seems likely that the majority of medical
assistance was carried out on a domestic level, with men treating
larger animals and women being responsible for smaller or younger
creatures.

---

[4] M. Pelling, 'Trade or Profession?', p. 232 and A. Wear, 'Religious Beliefs and Medicine
in Early Modern England', pp. 145–6.
[5] Guildhall Library, MS.5534 Farrier Court Journals, 1674, p. 1. pp. 2–4; H. Cook,
Decline, p. 20 and L. Prince, The Farrier and His Craft: The History of the Worshipful
Company of Farriers (London, 1980), pp. 1–2.

'Professional' versus Lay Healers in Early Modern England

The term 'professional' presents many difficulties, as the early modern definition is very clearly not the same as the modern one. Although there is relatively little disagreement about the modern definitions of 'professional' and 'lay' are in twenty-first century Britain, the situation is not so clear in the consideration of early modern practitioners. This is a topic that has long been of interest to academics, with the development of medicine simply being one component of the larger movements in the rise of professions in general.[6] According to David Coburn and Evan Willis, medicine is frequently used as an 'analytical example to advance theories of the professions' because 'it is assumed to be the epitome of what profession means'.[7] John Henry dates the beginnings of 'professionalism' of medicine to the Renaissance, pointing out that although medicine was established in late Middle Ages as one of the higher university faculties alongside theology and law, it only became professionalized through early modern licensing.[8]

I would argue that the requirement of governmental or other formal recognition through licensing is very much of a modern concept. If that argument were followed, then there would have been very few 'professional' medical healers in early modern England. These would have included physicians who were licensed by bishops, provincial medical guilds or the Royal College of Physicians or surgeons and midwives approved by bishops, companies or guilds.[9] In fact, there were numerous types of healers, many of which offered similar services that are not easily categorised. An early modern physician, for example, might have been university trained and licensed. However, there were even greater numbers of practitioners who used the title despite having no legal right to do so.[10] In other words, there was no assurance that an individual 'physician' had any qualifications, experience or even

---

[6] See, for example, T. Johnson, *Professions and Power* (London, 1972).

[7] D. Coburn and E. Willis, 'The Medical Profession: Knowledge, Power and Autonomy' in G.L. Albrecht, R. Fitzpatrick and S.C. Scrimshaw (eds) *The Handbook of Social Studies in Health & Medicine* (London, 2000), pp. 377–93.

[8] J. Henry, 'Doctors and healers: popular culture and the medical profession' in S. Pumfrey, P.L. Rossi and M. Slawinski (eds) *Science, culture and popular belief in Renaissance Europe* (Manchester, 1991), pp. 191–221.

[9] L.M. Beier, *Sufferers and Healers: The Experience of Illness in Seventeenth Century England* (London, 1987), p. 9.

[10] R. Porter, *Health for Sale: Quackery in England 1660–1850* (Manchester, 1989), p. 35.

knowledge. This story is the same for farriers, who might be called the equivalent of a physician in the world of animal health care.

Such examples suggest that it is only possible to use the most rudimentary categorisations when discussing early modern healers. There are inherent problems, however, in even determining what these should be. It is clear that modern definitions can not be used, as current terminology rests on highly regulated credentials and tests. On the other hand, contemporary terms must also be used carefully. For example, even a superficial examination of early modern texts illustrates the widespread use of derogatory labels such as 'quack' or 'mountebank'. In some cases these were levelled by so-called 'professional' practitioners such as members of the College of Physicians or members of the Farriers Company.[11] Even practitioners of astrological physick, who were often on the receiving end of such insults themselves, had no compunction about labelling others as 'ignorant Pretenders, which too frequently Quack about the city' and warning their own readers to 'loath Imposters and Quack-salving Knaves'. In fact, the widely published author of popular medical texts, William Salmon, who was regularly denounced as a quack, claimed that his long experience provided better qualifications than that of university educated men.[12]

Andrew Wear has suggested such sentiments were normal characteristics of a system of orthodox medicine where practitioners constantly claimed to know more than their competitors.[13] This is a logical conclusion, and one which can readily be viewed in the way in which modern biomedical and 'complementary' practitioners refer to each other in the media.[14] According to many sociologists, the reason for this hostility is due to the desire by biomedical physicians to protect what has been their 'monopoly...over the production and distribution of health care' in Britain.[15]

---

[11] J. Colbatch, *Four Treatises of Physick and Chirurgery* (London, 1698), p. xvi and Guildhall Library, MS 2890, *Ordinance Book*, seventeenth century, p. 29.

[12] R. Saunders, 1678, sig. B2r, T. Trigge, 1681, sig. A4v and W. Salmon, *Pharmacopoeia Londinensis. Or, the New London Dispensatory* (London, 1685), sig. A3r-v.

[13] A. Wear, 'Epistemology and Learned Medicine in Early Modern England' in D. Bates (ed.) *Knowledge and the Scholarly Medical Traditions* (Cambridge, 1995), p. 161.

[14] See, for example, M.A. Doel and J. Segrett, 'Self, Health, and Gender: complementary and alternative medicine in the British mass media', *Gender, Place and Culture*, 10, 2 (June 2003), 131–44.

[15] S. Harrison and W.I.U. Ahned, 'Medical Autonomy and the UK State 1975 to 2025' in S. Nettleton and U. Gustafsson (eds) *The Sociology of Health and Illness Reader* (Cambridge, 2002), pp. 310–21 and D. Greaves, *The Healing Tradition: Reviving the soul of Western Medicine* (Oxford, 2004), pp. 136–48.

Although a discussion of modern practitioners is outside the scope of this book, there is definitely a link between modern and early modern concerns about medical dominance and control. In veterinary medicine this is illustrated by the on-going efforts of members of the Company of Farriers to protect their trade.

Theoretically, they were the only men allowed to use the title as well as to be the only practising farriers in and within a seven-mile radius of London.[16] However, there is ample evidence that many others freely used the term themselves, either alone or in conjunction with phrases such as 'animal doctors'. Most of these healers would have gone through some type of formal or informal apprenticeship with someone who had worked with animals for many years. It seems likely that most would have agreed that 'Experience is the only probable means of success in any individual, whatever may be his profession.'[17]

Farriers

The hierarchy of animal practitioners matched that of the types of beasts they specialised in treating. This meant that the highest level was taken by those who worked with horses and held the legal right to be called a farrier and to treat horses in London. As members of the 'Company of Farriers' or 'Brotherhood of ffaryers', they practiced an Art and Trade ... of great antiquity... and of great use and benefitt to our Subjects for preserving of horses.[18] Their organisation had begun in 1356 as 'Marshalls of the city of London' in response to the 'many trespasses and grete damages' done by 'folk unwise .... [who] medill with Cures which they cannot bring to good ende'.[19]

The London company began in response to the 'many trespasses and grete damages' done by 'folk unwise which holde forges in the said Citie, and theym medill with Cures and which they cannot bring to good ende'.[20] In 1674 a Royal Charter made it a company, with the

---

[16] L.B. Prince, *The Farrier and His Craft. The History of the Worshipful Company of Farriers* (London, 1980), p.1.

[17] E. Snape, *Snape's Practical Treatise on Farriery* (London, 1791), p. iiii.

[18] Guildhall Library, MS.5534, *Farrier Court Journals*, 1674, p. 1.

[19] This was a corruption of the French 'mareschal' which is believed to have been used first in the mid-sixth century to refer to the keeper of the royal stables. A. Hyland, *The Medieval Horse* (Sutton, 1999), p. 51 and Guildhall Library, MS 2890, *Ordinance Book*, seventeenth century, p. 29.

[20] Guildhall Library, MS 2890, *Ordinance Book*, seventeenth century, p. 29.

power to search for defective works and medicines.[21] This was a very
elite institution with only forty-members, including a Master, three
wardens and 'not above twenty, nor under tenne assistants' in 1674. In
common with the College of Physicians, their members legally held a
monopoly in London and within a seven-mile radius.[22] Both laws were
widely ignored, threatening the respectability, collective security and
wealth of these men. The physician Daniel LeClerc complained about
quacks who 'endeavour to subvert the Honour and trample upon the
Dignity' of his profession. Such men, they argued, regularly destroyed
horses for 'want of due knowledge and skill in the right way of preserving of horses'.[23] Members of the Farriers Company had similar feelings
about those who:

> dayly come into this same Citie and fetche out horses of Innes and other
> houses…so that they [members of the Farrier's Company] be not nor can
> be able to lyf by there said craft.[24]

Such 'foreign' farriers were not the only risk to their trade, as the members of the Company of Farriers also faced competition from sources
closer to home. These included the many:

> unskillfull persons inhabiting within the Liberties of the said cities
> [London and Westminster] have of late taken upon them the said Art and
> Mistery, who have thereby for want of due knowledge and skill in the
> right way of preserving of horses destroyed many horses in or near the
> same cities.[25]

Although such a claim is impossible to substantiate, it is true that members of the Farriers Company were subject to a number of rules and
regulations. While they were not university educated, they were required
to undergo an apprenticeship 'by the space of sevene yeares at the least'
with an experienced farrier. Since members were allowed to take on
only three students at a time, each would have received a good deal of
personalised instruction.[26] Apprenticeships, a form of training which

---

[21] S.A. Hall, 'The State of the Art of Farriery in 1791', *Veterinary History*, New Series
7, 1 (January 1992), pp. 10–14.
[22] Guildhall Library, MS.5534 *Farrier Court Journals*, 1674, p. 1. pp. 2–4; H. Cook,
Decline, p. 20 and L. Prince, *The Farrier and His Craft: The History of the Worshipful
Company of Farriers* (London, 1980), pp. 1–2.
[23] Guildhall Library, MS. 2890, p. 41 and Guildhall Library, MS.5534, p. 1.
[24] D. LeClerc, *The History of Physick, or an Account of the Rise and Progress of the Art*
(London, 1699), sig. A2r and Guildhall Library, MS. 2890, p. 41.
[25] Idem, MS.5534, p. 1.
[26] Guildhall Library, MS.5534, p. 2

began in the middle ages, offered both social and economic advantages to young men. Firstly, it guaranteed that the boy would achieve at least a certain level of competence in treating animals. Secondly, it helped to control numbers of applicants, thereby preventing an excess of new farriers from entering the market.[27]

As farriery tended to be a family based trade, many prospective members, particularly by the Georgian period, served their apprenticeship under the supervision of a relative. The Snapes were unquestionably the most famous family of farriers, tending to succeeding generations of royal horses over the course of some two hundred years. Andrew Snape was royal farrier for Charles II, Robert, Richard and another Andrew Snape were other seventeenth-century members of the Farriers Company and Edward Snape was farrier to George III.[28] However, the majority of apprentices during the seventeenth century were not from London, and came from all over the country to learn their chosen trade.[29] The young men came from a variety of backgrounds, and few had fathers who were rural farriers. James Arneff, for example, was the son of a yeoman from Northumberland. This was also the case with Herbert Yapp from the 'city and country of Hereford'. Other apprentices had humbler origins. John Horneby was the son of the 'gardiner' at Barnard Castle in Durham. Henry Saxby was the son of a labourer from Northampton and Henry George's father was a taylor from Bedford.[30]

Although members of the Company of Farriers were at the top of the animal practitioner hierarchy, they were joined by a much larger group of men, both in London and the provinces, who were self-styled farriers. It seems likely that all offered similar services, which is hardly surprising given the etymology of the word 'farrier'. Originating with the Latin 'ferrarius' or 'ferrum', the term evolved into became 'ferrier' meaning one 'conversant in the working of iron' in Old French. As time

---

[27] J. Lane, 'The role of apprenticeship in eighteenth-century medical education in England' in W. Bynum and R. Porter (eds.) *William Hunter and the Eighteenth-Century Medical World* (Cambridge, 1985), pp. 57–105.

[28] J. Lane, 'Farriers in Georgian England' in A. Mitchell (ed.) *History of the Healing Professions*, Vol. III (Cambridge, 1993), pp. 99–117; E. Snape, *Snape's Practical Treatise on Farriery, &c.* (London, 1791), sig. A4r.; A. Snape, *The anatomy of a horse* (London, 1683), sig. A3r and Guildhall Library, MS.5534, p. 2.

[29] Relatively little information pertaining to the apprenticeship of farriers is currently available.

[30] Guildhall Library, London; MS. 5526, *Farrier's Company Apprentice Book*, seventeenth century, pp. 1, 65, 63, 64.

went by the definition became narrower, and by the sixteenth century blacksmiths produced iron horseshoes, which were fitted by farriers, who also provided medical care.[31]

The second most common title that men who treated horses would use was 'horseleech' or simply leech.[32] This term dates from the Middle Ages, when 'leech' was used to refer to all types of healers. It was not because they used leeches to draw blood, but was linked to the corruption of the old English word for healer, 'lece'.[33] Such men far outnumbered the membership of the Company of Farriers, and were the dominant animal healers in the countryside. Presumably, the level of stigma attached to these 'unqualified' practitioners was not as great as it would be today. There were vast numbers of horses in both town and country who would have required medical assistance. As David Harley has pointed out, consumers were seeking health, rather than a specific type of medical service.[34] In many cases, the expertise of the farrier or horse-leach would have been a more important consideration than any 'legal' qualifications that they might have had.

Lise Wilkinson has suggested that farriers and leeches 'were for the most part illiterate'.[35] This is a stereotypical statement that is unsupported by contemporary literature, which will be discussed in the following chapter. There were a large number of titles in which the author addressed his target audience of healers both within the introduction and the body of the text. Research conducted by Joan Lane has also shown found a great deal of evidence that both farriers and their apprentices could read and write in the mid eighteenth century.[36] Although there are no comparable studies for the previous century, there is no obvious reason for why this should not have also held true. Ideally, this theory could be tested through the study of surviving

---

[31] R. Ryder, *Animal Revolution: Changing Attitudes Towards Speciesism* (Oxford, 1989), pp. 53–4; K. Thomas, *Man and the Natural World*, pp. 153–4 and 166; F.R. Bell, 'The Days of the Farriers', *Veterinary History*, 9 (1977), pp. 3–6; Anon., *A Brief Examination of the Views of the Veterinary College* (London, 1795), p. 3; A. Adams, *The History of the Worshipful Company of Blacksmiths* (London, 1951), p. 34 and L. Prince, *The Farrier and His Craft. The History of the Worshipful Company of Farriers* (London, 1980), p. 3.

[32] W. Merrick, *The Classical Farrier* (London, 1788), p. iv and 'common farriers'.

[33] S. Pollington, *Leechcraft: Early English Charms, Plantlore and Healing* (Trowbridge, 2000), p. 41.

[34] D. Harley, 'The Good Physician and the Godly Doctor: The Exemplary Life of John Tylston of Chester (1663–1699), *The Seventeenth Century*, 9 (1994), p. 94.

[35] L. Wilkinson, *Animals and Disease*, p. 10.

[36] J. Lane, *Farriers in Georgian England*, p. 100.

business accounts and other records. Unfortunately, it has been impossible to locate such materials which could mean either that most farriers and leeches were unable to write, or simply that these materials have not survived over the centuries. At the very least, I would suggest that most London farriers and many rural horse-practitioners had at least a rudimentary knowledge of reading. As Wyn Ford has pointed out, a 'practical and pragmatic' literacy was a prerequisite for anyone needing to carry out everyday business matters.[37]

This argument is supported by the large number of vernacular medical and agricultural books addressed to 'farriers', 'horseleeches' or other types of leeches which offer indirect evidence that at least some of them could read.[38] For example, Leonard Mascall dedicated his book to farriers and horse-leeches who desired:

> The knowledge to help soreness and diseases in horses: They must well and perfectly understand of the present disease in the horse before they minister; also to look to him well, how many other griefs are growing on him ... also the operation of all such herbs and drugs as he doth minister unto them: with what quantity and portion of each thing thereof, and in what time and hour of the day and year is best.[39]

Although this sort of prescriptive advice does not necessarily translate into action, this quote suggests that the treatments administered by horseleeches paralleled those offered by members of the Company of Farriers. The same phenomenon was visible in human healthcare, whereby 'professional' practitioners offered the same types of services as the 'popular' healers.[40] The difference, presumably, is that the former did not have either the prerequisites or the desire necessary to join the Company of Farriers. Even so, because of the similarities of their work, horseleeches were more than entitled to refer to themselves as 'common farriers'.[41]

The continuing existence of such men also contradicts Robert Dunlop's accusation that animals were treated by 'individuals who mainly failed to

---

[37] W. Ford, 'The Problem of Literacy in Early Modern England', *History*, 76, 1993, p. 23.

[38] The existence of such books, however, does not prove that they were read by farriers or leeches.

[39] L. Mascall, *Cattle*, p. 97.

[40] D.E. Nagy, *Popular Medicine in Seventeenth-Century England* (Bowling Green, 1988), p. 3.

[41] S.A. Hall, 'The State of the Art of Farriery in 1791', *Veterinary History*, 7, 1992, pp. 10–11.

gain the respect of society'.[42] Although an animal owner might be willing to consult a healer once, they would only have continued to patronize him if they believed in and trusted his ability to care for their charges. The accounts of the Reverend John Crankanthorp, for example, included not one but a series of payments to 'one Marmaduke Feaks cowleech' for treating both his animals.[43] While itinerant farriers may have depended more on their ability to impress potential customers, local practitioners would have been most concerned with maintaining a good reputation. As William Winstanley pointed out, in some areas the most popular 'horse-doctor' commanded a virtual monopoly.[44] On the other hand if a farrier was known to be ineffective, or even cruel to his charges, he would be unable to attract or maintain any kind of a clientele.

Other Types of Healers

The term 'leech' was also used by practitioners who treated other types of 'cattel' or working animals. It appears that there was a hierarchy, albeit less formal, of these healers, starting with those who treated larger cattle such as 'ox-leeches' or 'cattle-leeches' down to the very low-liest 'cow-leeches' or 'cow-doctors'. According to contemporary authors, such men were in high demand, and were often asked to travel great distances to administer aid.[45] 'Lesser cattle', such as sheep, pigs and goats were more likely to be treated by the same agricultural workers or husbandmen who saw to their other daily needs. In most townships farmers would put their sheep into a 'common fold' looked after by one or two shepherds. Each farmer would provide enough hay for his animals, and one of the jobs of the shepherd was to allocate the food, pitch the fold and provide medical treatment for sick animals. There were also men called 'swineherds' who guarded and cared for herds of pigs while they were foraging in the forests.[46] Most pigs, except for those

---

[42] R.H. Dunlop and D.J. Williams, *Veterinary Medicine: An Illustrated History* (Chicago, 1996), p. 291.

[43] J. Crankanthorp, *Accounts of the Reverend John Crankanthorp of Fowlmere 1682–1710*, eds. P. Brassley, A. Lambert, P. Saunders (Cambridge, 1988), pp. 178–9 and 214.

[44] W. Winstanley, *The country-man's guide or plain directions for ordering.Curing. breeding choice, use and feeding. Of horses, cows, sheep, hoggs, &c* (London, 1679).

[45] J. Swaine, *Every Farmer his own Cattle-Doctor* (London, 1786), p. 1 and G. Markham, *Markhams Methode*, pp. 1–2, 50 and 30.

[46] E. Kerridge, The Sheepfold in Wiltshire and the Floating of the Watermeadows, *The Economic History Review* (1954), p 285 and J. Salisbury, *The Beast Within: Animals in the Middle Ages* (London, 1994), p. 27.

were used for breeding and some boars, were generally killed within the first year of life.[47] This might account for the relatively little amount of space dedicated to pigs in contemporary, popular veterinary texts.

As with farriers, there is little surviving direct evidence of the daily practices of cattle doctors or leeches. Unlike farriers, who specialised in horses, it seems likely that most of these men would not have focused exclusively on one type of animals, but would have treated many different ones. These healers would have needed to learn how to care for animals from others, probably in some sort of an informal apprenticeship. Leslie Pugh has tried to discredit these types of practitioners by calling them 'little more than herbalists' whose harmless though mainly ineffectual 'cures' were drawn from 'prescription books or collections of medical recipes'.[48] This is an interesting comment, given the continual accusations that such men would have been illiterate. As the following chapter illustrates, there were certainly veterinary texts that claimed to have been written for such readers. A number of texts begin with prefaces that complain of the lack of 'painful and labourious Oxeleech[es] or the tendency of 'unskilfull' animal healer to charge exorbitant fees.[49] However, before taking such statements at face value, it is necessary to think of the motivations that lay behind, namely the desire to convince potential purchasers that they would obtain better value from that book than from paying a leech.

This is not to suggest, however, that leeches were a homogeneous group of practitioners. While some may have practiced medicine full-time, there is ample evidence in primary sources that many more combined agricultural work with healing. John Clark, an agricultural labourer in Terling, was also referred to as a 'cowleech'. The accounts of the Reverend John Crankanthorp include a number of payments to another cowleech Marmaduke Feaks for treating both his red and his black cows.[50]

---

[47] J. Thirsk, 'Agricultural prices, wages, farm profits and rents' in J. Thirsk (ed)*The Agrarian History of England and Wales*, II (Cambridge, 1985), pp. 117–18; D. Hartley, *Food in England* (London, 1954), p. 101 and R. Malcolmson, and S. Mastoris, *The English Pig – A History* (London, 1998), pp. 14–15.

[48] L. Pugh, *Farriery to Veterinary*, p. 3.

[49] G. Markham, *Cavelarice, or the English Horseman* (London, 1607), *sig.* A2r and Harward, *The Herds-man's Mate*, sig. A3v.

[50] K. Wrightson and D. Levine, *Poverty and Piety in an English Village, Terling 1525–1700* (London, 1979), p. 23 and P. Brassley, A. Lambert and P. Saunders (eds.), *Accounts of the Reverend John Crankanthorp*, pp. 178–9 and 214.

Domestic Physick

> It shall be small profit to the husbandman to give his beast meat, and
> know not how to help & keep them in health & strength.[51]

It seems likely that the majority of treatments were actually administered by laymen at home, both for themselves and their animals.[52] Due
to their daily, close interaction with their animals, it seems likely that
many of these lay-healers would either have comparable or perhaps
even more experience than some part-time 'professional' healers. The
person most likely to treat human illness was likely to be the woman of
the house, or other female relatives. According to Gervase Markham,
knowledge of physick was one of the housewife's 'principal virtues'.
What we now call a 'healthy lifestyle', as well as 'primary health care'
would have been the responsibility of the female head of the family.[53]
As previously mentioned, it was also her role to look after the health of
smaller and weak animals. The care of horses and larger 'cattle', on the
other hand, was generally considered to be the responsibility of men.[54]

'Huswives' had a range of domestic duties which often involved extra
income or food for their families. Many of these tasks involved animals, particularly cows and chickens. Women were in charge of the
dairy and were expected to 'keep all under her jurisdiction' neat and
clean. This included managing any 'milkmaids' as well as seeing that
the animals were fed regularly. The housewife was also responsible for
rearing her calves 'upon the finger with floten milke' and tending to the
'cure of all diseases inclin'd to them'.[55]

Women also managed 'the ordering of poultry'. This included wrap-
ping poorly chicks in wool and putting them near the fire. According to
Gervase Markham, 'pullen' loved the 'aire of the fire' as they found the
smell to be 'delightful'. Another text suggested that the fire be scented

---

[51] L. Mascal, *Cattle*, p. 5.

[52] R. Trow-Smith, *A History of British Livestock Husbandry to 1700* (London, 1957),
p. 240.

[53] A.W. Sloan, *English Medicine*, p. 8; G. Markham, *The English Housewife 1615*, ed.
M. Best (London, 1994), p. 8; M. Pelling, 'Thoroughly Resented? Older Women and the
Medical Role in Early Modern London' in L. Hunter and S. Hutton (eds.) *Women,
Science and Medicine 1500–1700* (Thrupp, 1997), p. 70 and W. Salmon, *Salmon's Family
Dictionary, or Household Companion* (London, 1702), sig. A3r.

[54] L. Mascal, *Cattle*, sig. A2r.

[55] G. Markham, *A way to get wealth* (London, 1648), p. 193; J.S. *The accomplished
ladies rich closet of rarities* (London, 1687), p. 146 and R. Shoemaker, *Gender in English
Society 1650–1850* (Harlow, 1998), p. 182.

with rosemary, and advised that 'it is proper to keep them a Fortnight in the House, before you suffer them to goe abroad'.[56] It seems likely that women would also have nursed small, young animals within the household.[57]

As with most types of lay-healers, women would have obtained their medical knowledge both from the oral and the print tradition. In most cases, this probably included watching and working alongside their mother, or senior female in their household. It seems likely that both female and male laypeople utilized the same types of medical publications that practitioners did, in addition to acquiring information orally or through manuscript sources including recipe or household books or correspondence.[58] Husbandry books generally contained a great deal of veterinary advice, which would have been of use to husbandmen, small farmers, shepherds, swineherds, herdsmen and other agricultural workers. As one contemporary author pointed out, it was important to know how to 'apply [medicines] to himselfe, whereas neither 'Physician nor Apothecarie can bee had'.[59] The same consideration would have been true for the animals that such people owned and/or cared for.

Male lay-healers, who cared for the health of the majority of animals, fall into such a huge category that it is an impossible task to draw blanket conclusions about their training or knowledge. Most were likely to have worked regularly with animals in some capacity or another, giving them an intimate knowledge of their habits and behaviour. As a result, it seems probable that such carers were likely to provide medical attention much quicker and perhaps more effectively, than a leech who treated all types of animal. They also would be likely to know the history of the animal, including their tendency to suffer from certain disorders and how they responded to treatments in the past.

A shepherd, for example, was responsible protecting his flocks, and his dog, from the 'injuries of the elements'.[60] According to one writer,

---

[56] G. Markham, *A way to get wealth*, p. 152 and A. S., *The husbandman, Farmer, and Grasier's Compleat* Instructor (London, 1697), p. 150.

[57] D. Simonton, *A History of European Women's Work 1700 to the Present* (London, 1998), p. 20 and H. Barker, 'Women and Work' in H. Barker and E. Chalus (eds) *Women's History, 1700–1850* (Abingdon, 2005), 124–152.

[58] For example, Buckinghamshire Records Office, *Book of Receipts* – Chequers Mss D138/16/6/1, late 17th century and Anon., *English Farrier*, sig. A2r.

[59] O. Wood, *An Alphabetical Book of Physicall Secrets* (London, 1639), sig. A2v.

[60] T. Tryon, *The country-man's companion: or, A New Method of Ordering Horses & Sheep So as to preserve them both from diseases and casualties* (London, 1688) p. 70.

he had three main duties: 'first for their food; secondly for their fold; and thirdly, for their health'.[61]

This included steering them away from danger, moving to new pastures to avoid rot and finding a dry resting place. A major part of their job would have included the provision of both preventative and remedial medicine. The former included covering the sheep with a thick salve (the forerunner of sheep dig) in the autumn to guard them against lice and scab, as well as protecting them from the weather. They would also be responsible for castrating the males, after which they would dress the wound with a mixture of herb butter, molten tallow or tar. [62]

A shepherd would also have been familiar with preventative and remedial medicine for his dog. According to John Caius, there were three main types of 'Englishe dogges':

> A gentle kinde, seruing the game.
> A homely kind, apt for sundry necessary vses.
> A currishe kinde, méete for many toyes.[63]

Although pet dogs were very popular during the Tudor and Stuart periods, most were expected to carry out some type of work. Some were used to pull carts, sleds or ploughs while many others were used for tracking specific types of animals, with certain dogs bred to hunt 'buck, bear, bull and boar' and others the 'hare, coney and hedghog'.[64] Dogs were also called upon to carry out a range of other duties, from guarding animals or humans, to entertaining the latter by dancing to music to turning the wheel of a kitchen spit for roasting meat.[65]

Joanna Swabe has argued that dogs 'historically received very little formal veterinary attention because they weren't important economically, were of little threat to human health and were easily replaceable'.[66] This is a problematic statement, negated by the vast amount of information on health care for dogs in popular veterinary texts. Secondly, dogs were valued for many reasons and fulfilled a variety of different

---

[61] E. Toppsell, *The Historie of Foure-Footed Beastes* (London, 1607), p. 467.

[62] M.L. Ryder, *Sheep and man* (London, 1983), pp. 479–480.

[63] J. Caius, *Of Englishe dogges* (London, 1576), p. 2

[64] Anon, *A treatise of oxen, sheep, hogs and dogs with their natures, qualities and uses* (London, 1683), p. 43.

[65] J. Caius, *Dogges*, p. 35.

[66] J. Swabe, 'Veterinary dilemmas: ambiguity and ambivalence in human-animal interaction' in A.L. Poderscek, E.S. Paul, J.A. Serpell (eds) *Companion Animals and Us* (Cambridge, 2000), 292–311.

roles in early modern society. These included 'grey-hounds, blood-hounds, sluth-hounds, gaze-hounds, spaniels, tumbers, beagles, bear-dogs, house-dogs [ie guard dogs] tarriers, harriers' and many other breeds. There were also dogs known as 'comforters' which were the modern equivalent of a household pet.[67] Edward Toppsell expressed the sentiments of many people when he wrote that 'there is not any creature without reason, more loving to his Master, nor more service-able then is a dog'.[68] Although I have been unable to find any references to sick dogs being treated by a leech, I would suggests that this meant that they would have been subject to the ministrations of whoever saw to their diet and daily care.

The same holds true for pigs, of whom it was said that 'there are few beasts more subject to distempers than the Swine'. There do not seem to have been any swine-leeches or other specialists in their treatment. This may well have been that with the exception of breeding sows and some boars, most pigs were killed by the end of their first year of life. That said, if they were ill it is likely that they would have either have been cared for by a swineherd, or perhaps the husbandman. Gervase Markham was uncharacteristically economic with words when he described the role of the swineherd. In general, this consisted of 'the preservation of swine' through the proper government of their behav-iour and ensuring that the received enough food. They were also responsible for whatever medical attention the animals might need as a result of 'Colds or Coughs, Belly-Ach, Lameness, Diseases in the Gall and Flux', which they were subject to.[69]

Conclusion

> The Righteous Man (saith the inspired Prophet) is Merciful to his Beast: Which Mercy, Compassion or Pitifulness consists not only in his not abusing them with excessive Labour, and unreasonable Stripes and Hardships, but in providing for them convenient Food, and helping to free them of Diseases or Infirmities.[70]

---

[67] A.S., *The husbandman, Farmer, and Grasier's Compleat Instructor* (London, 1697), pp. 131–134.

[68] E. Toppsell, *The Historie*, p. 110.

[69] G. Markham, *A way to get wealth*, p. 128; R. Maclcolmson and S. Mastoris, *The English Pig: A History* (London, 1998), p. 14 and Anon., *The Experienced Jockey, Compleat Horseman; or Gentlemans Delight* (London, 1684), p. 326.

[70] T. Tryon, *The country-man's companion* (London, 1688), sig. A2r.

There were many people involved in the health care of sick animals in early modern England. As with human medicine, there was a comparable hierarchy of healers within the commonly accepted model of 'the medical marketplace'. Although it has long been a commonplace that animals would have to rely on ministrations carried out by erstwhile 'human' healers, the historical evidence proves otherwise. There was, in fact, a highly complex system of animal health care which involved healers who specialised in horses, as well as a broader range of practitioners who would treat almost any type of 'cattle'.

Unlike elite physicians, these men and women would either have learned their healing skills through a formal or informal apprenticeship, often supplemented by popular veterinary texts. Some of these services could be purchased or bartered for in the marketplace, as well as those that were available 'free of charge'. The main categories of animal healers consisted of 'professional' farriers, self-styled farriers, horseleeches and horse-doctors and leeches specialising in other types of working animals. Members of the Company of Farriers were at the top of the hierarchy and, in theory, enjoyed a monopoly on treating horses in and within a seven mile radius of London. The second level also consisted of men who practiced horse medicine without the benefit of belonging to such an elite organisation. They sometimes referred to themselves as farriers even though they were not legally entitled to do so, while others were known as horseleeches or horse-doctors. There were also a variety of practitioners further down the scale who treated lowlier animals, such as cows or sheep. Depending on their speciality, they might treat the 'oxe, bull, cowe, or calfe' who were 'beasts naturally of a slow and heavie disposition, yet fit for draught'.[71] Many were also referred to as leeches, although some preferred to use titles such as 'cow-doctor'.

The largest category of medical providers, however, fall under the heading of 'lay-healers'. It seems likely that the majority were men who spent much of their time with animals, either as husbandmen or as shepherds, swineherds, herds-men, grooms or other types of agricultural workers. I would argue that the medical care they provided would often have been superior to that offered by 'professional' animal healers, particularly those who treated all types. After all, those who lived

---

[71] J. Swabe, *The Burden of Beasts*, p. 71 and G. Markham, *Markhams Methode*, pp. 1–2, 50 and 30.

and worked alongside their charges would have been able to offer the quickest assistance based on an intimate and long-term knowledge of their general health and propensity to fall ill.

Judging by the breakdown of work in texts such as Gervase Markham's *The Way to Get Wealth*, men were more likely to look after larger and/ or older animals. Women, on the other hand, would have been in charge of the cows in their dairy and the poultry in their henhouses. These were both very important roles in the economy of their households, with the animals producing both for home consumption and, perhaps, for sale in the market. There is also evidence that women nursed other small or young animals.

Unfortunately, little direct evidence of the medical care offered by laypeople has survived. However, there is little question that people did provide care for their sick animals in order to protect their valuable and prized possessions. There is also a great deal of indirect proof about the ways in which people provided their animals with health care. The following chapter will discuss the evolution of veterinary literature from the earliest known manuscripts through the seventeenth century. This will be followed in the third section by an in-depth examination of the types of preventative and remedial veterinary treatments that were available in early modern England.

CHAPTER FOUR

THE PRINT CULTURE AND VETERINARY MEDICINE

> Amongst many temporall [sic] Benefits which Divine Bounty hath in severall ages manifested to mankinde [sic] the invention of the Mystery, of Art of Printing may rightly be acknowledged one of the greatest, as an exact and exquisite Instrument, opening to the understanding, not onley [sic] all naturall Sciences, but even supernaturall [sic] Mysteries.[1]

As the previous chapter illustrated, there were a large number of people involved in the health care of in domesticated animals who were unable to fend for themselves.[2] There were a variety of medical options available, many of which could be purchased in the medical marketplace, while others were available by bartering or for free. The hierarchy of animal practitioners began with members of the Company of Farriers, followed by a range of what might now be called 'non-professional' healers. In common with human health care, it seems likely that in most cases the initial, and sometimes only medical intervention, would be that administered in a domestic setting by lay-healers.

There were many ways in which both 'professional' and 'non-professional' healers could have gained their medical knowledge. Before the advent of mechanical printing in the late fifteenth century most medical information would have been disseminated through the oral culture. Peter Murray Jones has suggested that prior to 1375 the relatively small numbers of manuscript texts being produced would have been mainly used by one of two groups. The first were university students, followed by the somewhat amorphous 'highly educated readers'. Animal practitioners, of course, would automatically have been excluded from the first category and were unlikely to fall into the latter. There were also a number of Middle English manuscripts either written for or owned by highly trained physicians, joined by a number of

---

[1] W. Ball, *A Briefe Treatise Concerning the Regulating of Printing* (London, 1651), sig. A3r.

[2] S. Budiansky, *The Covenant of the Wild: Why Animals Chose Domestication* (New York, 1992), p. 123.

vernacular 'lower level' medical texts in the later part of the middle-ages, which might have been used by veterinary practitioners.[3]

The development of printing dramatically transformed the way in which all types of medical knowledge could be transmitted and disseminated. For the first time, large numbers of identical images could be produced quickly and cheaply and distributed nationally. Topics such as health, medicine and diet proved to be particularly popular and resulted in a wide range of publications which targeted all segments of the literate public. By the seventeenth century, such works had become one of the most profitable segments of the western European publishing trade.[4]

The relationship between the print culture and medical beliefs and practices has been the topic of growing interest to academics over the past few decades. A number of studies have suggested that the print culture had a major impact on contemporary medical beliefs and practices in every stratum of early modern English society.[5] However, in common with most modern works on medical beliefs and practices during this period, the discussions focus almost exclusively on human health care. This is hardly surprising, given the generally anthropocentric attitudes about early veterinary history in general. However, it is a grave oversight, as the wealth of contemporary English language works on animal health care provides the strongest evidence and examples of veterinary beliefs and practices in the early modern period.

---

[3] P.M. Jones, 'Medicine and Science', in L. Hellinga and J.B. Trapp (eds) *The Cambridge History of the Book in Britain*, III (Cambridge, 1991), p. 433 and L.E.Voigts and M.R. McVaugh, 'A Latin Technical Phlebotomy and Its Middle English Translation', *Transactions of the American Philosophical Society*, New Ser., Vol 74, 2 (1984) 1–69.

[4] P. Burke, *Popular Culture in Early Modern Europe*, second edition (Aldershot, 1994), p. 250 and W.D. Smith, *Consumption and the Making of Respectability, 1600–1800* (London, 2002), p. 124.

[5] See, for example L.E. Voigts, 'Scientific and Medical Books' in J. Griffiths and D.A. Pearsall (eds.) Book production and publishing in Britain 1375–1475 (Cambridge, 1989), pp. 345–402; M. Fissell, 'Readers, Texts, and Contexts: Vernacular medical works in early Modern England' in R. Porter (ed.) *The Popularization of Medicine 1650–1850* (London, 1992); P. Isaac, 'Pills and Print' in R. Harris and M. Myers (ed.) *Medicine, Mortality and the Book Trade* (Folkestone, Kent, 1998) 25–49; P.M. Jones, 'Medicine and science' , 433–49; A. Wear, *Knowledge & Practice in English Medicine, 1550–1680* (Cambridge, 2000), esp. 40–45; E.L. Furdell, *Publishing and Medicine in Early Modern England* (Rochester, 2002); A. Johns, 'Science and the Book' in J. Barnard and D.F.M. McKenzie (eds) *The Cambridge History of the Book*, IV 1557–1695 (Cambridge, 2002), 274–303; G.R. Keiser, 'Two Medieval Plague Treatises and Their Afterlife in Early Modern England', *Journal of the History of Medicine and Allied Sciences*, 58 (July, 2003), 292–324 and L. Hill Curth, *English Almanacs, astrology and popular medicine, 1550–1700* (Manchester, 2007).

This chapter will discuss the two main categories of such publications produced in early modern England, roughly divided into books and ephemeral literature. It will begin with a brief overview of the evolution of veterinary literature from the times of the 'ancients' to the advent of the printing press in the late fifteenth century. This will be followed by a section on early printed medical literature, both that which focused on animals as well as works which incorporated animal health care alongside that for humans. The third section will look at 'ephemeral' literature which discussed animal health care. Its major focus will be on the veterinary content of cheap, annual almanacs, which were the first true form of mass media in Europe. Finally, the chapter will conclude by briefly discussing the issues of literacy and whether the kind of target animal healers such works were aimed at were likely to have been able to actually use them.

Veterinary Literature before Printing

There is some debate as to the age of the oldest surviving veterinary text. In his overview of veterinary medicine, Denis Karasszon has suggested that the earliest was written in Chaldea over 3,400 years ago. That said, the date has been taken from a copy translated around 710 A.D. as the original no longer exists. Sir Frederick Smith, the author of the magisterial, three volume series on the history of veterinary literature, thought otherwise. Based on a series of articles published in the *Journal of Comparative Pathology and Therapeutics* between 1912 and 1918, Smith aimed to 'trace the history of veterinary literature from the earliest known times down to the middle of the nineteenth century'. Smith argued that technically the very first texts were the Laws of Hammurabi (c. 2100 B.C.), which referred to veterinary practitioners. However, he attributed the first veterinary textbook to be that written by Democritus of Abdera (470–402 B.C.) and Simon of Athens (430 B.C.).[6]

The fifth century B.C. is generally considered to be a very important period in the growth of medicine, with the second half experiencing the 'birth' of both medical literature and 'the art of medicine'. This is linked to the work of Hippocrates of Cos, referred to as 'the Father of

---

[6] D. Karasszon, *A Concise History of Veterinary Medicine*, (trans) E. Farkas (Budapest, 1988), pp. 13 and 94–5 and F. Smith, *The Early History of Veterinary Literature*, I (London, 1919, reprinted 1976), pp. 5–7.

Medicine'. Although very little is known about the man, his fame is due to the sixty to seventy medical texts referred to as the *Hippocratic Corpus*, with a particular emphasis on the Hippocratic Oath. Vivian Nutton has described the collection as being based on the 'psychological, moral and philosophical role' that sickness played in society, rather than on the phenomenon itself.[7] *De natura hominis*, for example, introduced the theory of the four humours. Although the Hippocratic writers focused on human health, their knowledge of internal functions was based on animal dissections. As a result, some of the material found in *De natura hominis* provided the core of Aristotle's *Historia animalium*. Written in the fourth century B.C., this text divided animals into eight genera, which were 'scientific extensions' of categories like birds or fish. Each of these was then separated into species which shared similar physical traits. The work did not, however, discuss examples of healthy or diseased states in the creatures.[8]

Aristotle (c. 384–322 B.C.) is often credited about being 'the most important of the philosophers' on nature and the status of animals. With a keen interest in what we would now call biology and zoology, Aristotle gathered a range of information on various animals, birds and fish which led him to formulate the 'Scala Naturae' theory 'Ladder of Nature'. This was a hierarchical structure which placed humans at the peak with animals and plants at various levels below according to their reasoning abilities.[9]

Unlike the Hippocratic Corpus, many ancient veterinary manuscripts have only survived in fragmentary form. Fortunately, much of their original content has survived thanks to its integration into later works. These include authors such Cato who wrote about the care and management of animals in the third century B.C. Marcus Tarentus Varro's (116–27 B.C.) *Concerning Agriculture* covered topics from farm buildings to the care of animals, including sheep, pigs, birds, fowls and bees. He divided their diseases into two categories, those for which 'medici' had to be summoned and those that could be dealt with by the

---

[7] V. Nutton, *Ancient Medicine*, (London, 2004), p. 51–53.

[8] J. Jouana, 'The Birth of Western Medical Art' in M. Grmek (ed) *Western Medical Thought from Antiquity to the Middle Ages* (London, 1998), pp. 22–71; R. Porter, *The Greatest Benefit to Mankind: A Medical History of Humanity from Antiquity to the Present* (London, 1997). p. 56 and D. Depew, 'Humans and Other Political animals in Aristotle's History of Animals', *Phronesis*, 40, 2, 1995 , pp. 156–181.

[9] V. Nutton, *Ancient Medicine* (London, 2004), p. 118 and J. Serpell, In the Company of Animals: A study of human-animal relationships (Cambridge, 1996), p. 15.

owner or caretaker.[10] Columella was a later, Roman writer whose work failed to survive in full. Based on knowledge gained in his travels, his *Husbandry*, which is thought to have been finished around 55 A.D., contains medical observations on horses and various types of cattle.[11]

Thanks to Vegetius (5th c AD), who is often lauded as 'the father of veterinary medicine', the work of these and other early veterinary writers has survived. Some historians have argued that this title should not be given to someone who 'merely' compiled ancient and contemporary veterinary writings. Vegetius' compilation explained the important role that hygiene played in animal health care, as well as discussing how to diagnose and treat a wide range of diseases in horses and other types of working animals.[12] The question of where this material was gathered from seems less important than the fact that it did appear to have a major impact on later authors, including those living in what became known as the Byzantine Empire.

In 395 A.D. the old Roman Empire was divided into Eastern and Western segments, each with their own emperor. Rome was the capital of the former, and Constantinople, or what had previously been Byzantium, for the latter. The 'Byzantine Empire' gradually became the centre for medical learning and innovation with a range of scholars interested in reworking and reinterpreting Galen's texts. In addition, there was a growing interest in new forms and types of medicinal ingredients and treatments.[13] The fourth and fifth centuries were also a period of on-going border fighting on horses between the cavalry and barbarians. As a result, the main interest in veterinary medicine seems to have been on treating sick or wounded horses who played a major role in warfare.[14]

The best known contemporary text was the *Hippiatrica* (c. fifth or sixth century A.D.) an encyclopedic collection of excerpts from seven

---

[10] J.N. Adams, *Pelagonius and Latin Veterinary Terminology in the Roman Empire* (Leiden, 1995), p. 72.

[11] F. Smith, *Veterinary*, Vol. I, pp. 14–15.

[12] F.R. Vegetius, *The foure bookes of Flavius Renatus Vegetius* (trans) J. Sadler (London, 1572), sig C1v; L. Wilkinson, 'Veterinary cross-currents in the history of ideas on infectious diseases', *Journal of the Royal Society of Medicine*, 73 (November 1980), 818–826 and F. Smith, *Veterinary Literature*, I, pp. 26–7.

[13] M. Grmek. 'Medicine in the Byzantine and Arab Worlds' in M. Grmek (ed) *Western Medical Thought from Antiquity to the Middle Ages* (London, 1988), pp. 139–169.

[14] J. Scarborough, 'Introduction', *Symposium on Byzantine Medicine*, Dumbarton Oaks Papers, Vol 38, (London, 1984), ix–xvi and D. Karasszon, *Veterinary*, p. 111.

Late Antique veterinary manuals. The *Hippiatrica* was a vast work which focused on practical treatments, organized by ailments and appropriate recipes. Many of the symptoms and diseases described, such as lameness, cough, colic, laminitis and parasites still affect horses today. It also included a variety of other information, including how to breed, break, feed, groom and stable horses. A recent book by Anne McCabe suggests that the earliest material found in the work can be traced to the 14th century B.C. cuneiform found at Ras Shamra-Ugarit in Syria.[15] As with large numbers other early texts, the *Hippiatrica* is known from later, rather than contemporary copies. The popularity of this text is illustrated by the numerous copies that were produced throughout the sixth, seventh and succeeding centuries and distributed throughout France, Germany, Italy, the Netherlands and England.[16]

The commonest of all illustrated manuscripts (other than Bibles) in the Romanesque and Gothic Middle Ages were said to be 'bestiaries' or books of beasts. It is thought that the earliest surviving copy dates from the 8 or 9th century B.C.[17] In England, bestiaries were said to have 'reached their apogee' during the first half of the thirteenth century. Although the content differs between surviving manuscripts, in general, 'books of beasts' were based on the *Physiologus* written sometime between the second and fourth centuries A.D., with later chapters added about additional animals and birds. Although these were not veterinary texts, they are important for the types of entries they contained, generally broken down by type of animal. The majority began with an explanation of the name of an animal, followed by an illustration of the beast in question. Horses, for example, were said to get their Latin name 'equi' because 'when they are harnessed in a team of four, they are equally matched'.[18]

The next major work on veterinary medicine also dates from the twelfth century, or what Denis Karasszon refers to as the 'age of chivalry'. Although the death of horses during war was an on-going problem, he suggests that the losses reached unprecedented numbers during the Crusades of 1228–9. This was said to have led to Frederick II

---

[15] A. McCabe, *A Byzantine Encyclopedia of Horse Medicine: The Sources, Compilation, and Transmission of the Hippicatrica* (Oxford, 2007), pp. 1, 2–4 and 15.

[16] F. Smith, *Veterinary*, Vol. I, pp. 42–3.

[17] W. George and B. Yapp, *The Naming of Beasts: Natural history in the medieval bestiary* (London, 1991), pp. 2–3.

[18] J.E. Salisbury, *The Beast Within: Animals in the Middle Ages* (New York, 1994), pp. 114–117 and R. Barber, *Bestiary* (Woodbridge, 1999) pp. 1–12 and 101.

instructing his mareschal Giordano Rufo (alternatively referred to as Ruffus, Russo or Russo) to produce *Medicina Eqorum* in 1250. There was relatively new material in this work which was based on 'observation, tradition and analogy' mixed with 'practical therapy'. Although the original has not survived, many of the numerous copies have, including versions in Latin, Italian, Sicilian, German, French and one in Hebrew.[19]

According to Frederick Smith, the oldest surviving, original veterinary manuscript actually produced in England was the Anglo-Normon *Medicinale Anglicum*. It was also referred to as the *Leech Book*, a phrase that continued to appear in medieval manuscripts with 'leech' referring to the early English word for healer. The copy at the British Library contains three volumes and focuses more heavily on diseases and injuries in humans than animals. It seems more accurate to label the thirteenth century Norman-French text on husbandry by Walter de Henley as the oldest veterinary manuscript produced in England.[20]

Before 1375 most medical books used in Britain were linked to study of medicine in universities. The majority were written in Latin, some in Greek and almost none in English. Major changes began to appear over the next century, when public demand resulted in a number of medical manuscripts being translated into Middle English and Anglo-Norman. Since the majority are compilations of earlier works, most could not be said to have an author, in the modern definition of the word. In many cases, it is also not possible to identify an editor or compiler. It seems likely that many were put together by anonymous medieval religious clerics in Latin. However, the rising demand for translation of such manuscripts, apparent by the late fourteenth century, suggests that some could have been produced by less formally educated scribes.[21]

During the fifteenth century, the growing number of medical manuscripts included many veterinary texts that were produced in Europe. The majority were compilations of earlier writers such as Hippocrates, Vegetius and Johannes Rufus. Frederick Smith dryly remarked that

---

[19] D. Karasszon, *Veterinary*, pp. 175–8 and F. Smith, *Veterinary*, Vol I, p. 78.

[20] British Library, MSS 12 D. XVII *LÆCEBOC*; S. Pollington, *Leechcraft: Early English Charms, Plant lore and Healing* (Trowbridge, 2000), p. 41 and O. Cockayne, *Leechdoms, Wortcunning and Starcraft of Early England* (London, 1865).

[21] P.M. Jones, 'Medicine and science', pp. 433–4; P.M. Jones, 'Image, Word, and Medicine in the Middle Ages' in J.A. Givens, K.M. Reeds, A. Touwaide (ed) *Visualizing Medieval Medicine and Natural History, 1200–1550* (Aldershot, 2006), 1–24 and F.N.L. Poynter, *The Evolution of Medical Practice in Britain* (London, 1961), p. 118.

very few of these works were written in England for the reason that 'there was nothing produced worthy of the process'. He went on to list several such manuscripts before dismissing them for illustrating that 'no progress beyond mediocrity' was made during this period.[22] Such a comment is hardly surprising, given his general attitude towards the quality of historical veterinary works. As the following section will show, large number of these 'mediocre' works continued to form the core of the newly printed manuals that began to appear in the late fifteenth century.

The Print Culture and Veterinary Literature

> Yea, Printing puts Books into everymans hand, whereby though we cannot practice all things, we may try all things.[23]

Frederick Smith credited the invention of the mechanical printing press as marking 'the end of ignorance' in veterinary literature.[24] Such a dramatic statement is somewhat surprising given the fact that the majority of early printed books were simply translations of earlier manuscripts which were also compilations of earlier writings. Ian Green has suggested that the English print trade began in the late fifteenth century for the purpose of reducing the high cost of handwritten texts.[25] This could well have been one, although probably not the only reason. The printing process also allowed the mass reproduction of precisely the same text, which was repeatable on subsequent occasions and in different locations.[26] Prefaces to the readers, and other textual evidence, suggests that many targeted both 'professional' and lay animal healers, a topic which will be discussed in the following section.

Ian Maclean has suggested that there were three major periods of development for European printed books which contained medical content. Although he bases this exclusively on texts about human health, his categories apply just as well to those for animals.[27] Maclean's first

---

[22] F. Smith, *Veterinary*, Vol. I, pp. 107 and 121.

[23] Anon., *A Brief discourse concerning printing and printers* (London, 1663), p. 22.

[24] F. Smith, *Veterinary*, p.121.

[25] I. Green, *Print and Protestantism in Early Modern England* (Oxford, 2000), p. 12.

[26] A. Johns, *The Nature of the Book: Print and Knowledge in the Making* (Chicago, 1998).

[27] I. Maclean, *Logic, Signs and Nature*, pp. 37–8 and P. Slack, 'Mirrors of Health', pp. 240–2.

period was from the late fifteenth century up until around 1525. Although Padua produced the largest number of medical texts in the 1470's, by the 1490's Venice began to be known as the centre of medical, academic and professional publishing. The majority of these texts consisted of folio editions in Italian which followed the form and style of medieval manuscripts produced by clerics on herbs and health regimes.[28]

A similar trend is evident in the vernacular veterinary texts printed during this period. The first work on horsemanship appeared in Spain in 1495, followed by three Italian publications in 1499, 1517 and 1518.[29] In England the thirteenth century manuscript *Boke of Husbandrie* by Walter de Henley was published first in 1508, followed by a number of similar versions (often under a different author's name) throughout the following century. The earliest version was a short, fairly generalized text on farm-related topics. What little advice it contained on animal care was quite elementary such as that 'plough bestes' should be given enough food to allow them to 'sustene theyr labour' or that 'theyr stable be made cleane every day'.[30] Later, greatly expanded versions of *The Boke of Husbandry* contained a wide range of advice on health care, despite his apology for not having the space 'to shew medicines & remedies' for all 'diseases and sorances' the text does address a number of illness in horses, sheep and other cattle [ie working animals].[31]

The earliest printed edition of the *Hippiatrica* appeared in Paris in 1530, around the same time that Vegetius's work was published in Basle. This was followed in 1546 by a Venetian version of Girolamo Fracastoro's comparative treatise on the similarities between infections of contagious diseases in humans and animals according to Galenic and astrological principles.[32] In the early part of the twentieth century, Sir Frederick Smith had suggested that the first veterinary book was printed in England between 1510 and 1525. However, when Smith's impressive three volume history of early modern veterinary was updated in the mid 1970's, this specific text could not be located. The sole known edition of *Mediciues for Horses*, held at Trinity College

---

[28] L. Hellinga, 'Medical Incunabula' in R. Myers and M. Harris (eds.) *Medicine, Mortality and the Book Trade* (Winchester, 1998), p. 77.

[29] J. Thirsk, *The Rural Economy of England* (London, 1984), p. 389.

[30] W. De Henley, *The Boke of Husbandrie*. (London, 1503), sig. 8v and 9r.

[31] J. Fitzherbert, *The Boke of Husbandry* (London, 1533), sig. F1r.

[32] F. Smith, Vol. I, p. 42–3 and L Wilkinson, 'Veterinary cross-currents in the history of ideas on infectious diseases', *Journal of the Royal Society of Medicine*, 73 (November 1980), 818–826.

Cambridge, is now thought to have been printed around 1565. It may well be, however, that an earlier version of this work will be rediscovered in the future.[33]

Maclean's second period ran from 1525 until 1565, which marked the appearance of a growing number of new books on astrology, alchemy and new diseases which appeared alongside more scholarly Latin and Greek versions. Translations also continued to be popular, with about one third of popular sixteenth century titles originating from either older Greek or foreign language texts. In fact, it has been estimated that reprints of works first published before 1558 made up around 1/3 of the total output of medical books during the second half of the century.[34] As with earlier texts, the majority of these were either compilations and/or re-workings of earlier works, although some claimed to be 'supplemented' by the author's own experience.

The final period in Maclean's categorisation was from 1565 to 1625. This was said to be a 'golden period' which included the development of the Frankfurt Book Fair. That said, although European fairs which attracted book dealers also took place in Lyons and Leipzig, few Englishmen were thought to attend. Unlike university educated physicians, many animal practitioners were not likely to have been interested in foreign language veterinary texts. Potential lay-readers would also, presumably, have preferred books written in the vernacular.

As previously mentioned, many texts were translated into English while a growing number were produced by English writers as a 'service' to their fellow countrymen. One of the earliest was Thomas Blundeville's *Fowre Chiefest Offices Belonging to Horsemanshippe* was initially published in 1566. The fact that it became the 'most reprinted popular text of the sixteenth century' suggests that there was a great demand for that sort of work.[35] In 1585 Leonard Mascall produced a book on the care 'poultrie and other foule' which he claimed was 'such as hath not here before bene written, or revealde in our english tongue'. Two years later he followed with a text on the care or 'government for our most used

---

[33] F. Smith, *Veterinary*, Vol. I, pp 142–4.

[34] P.M. Jones, 'Medicine and Science' p. 434 and H.S. Bennett, *English Books and Readers 1558 to 1603* (Cambridge, 1965), p. 181.

[35] K. Raber, 'Nation and Race in Horsemanship Treatises' in K. Raber and T.J. Tucker (eds) *The Culture of the Horse: Status, Discipline and Identity in the Early Modern World* (Basingstoke, 2005), 225–243.

cattell, as oxen, kinde, calves, horses, sheepe, hogges, and such: with divers approved remedies for them.[36]

It is somewhat surprising that Maclean's categorization ends in the second half of the 1620's, shortly before the virtual explosion in popular print. From nearly the beginning of mechanical printing until 1640 the book industry had been controlled through a partnership of king, state and church. The collapse of censorship in the 1640's resulted in a flood of all sorts of publications including those on human and veterinary medicine.[37]

John Crawshey was one of the most popular seventeenth century writers to discuss the health of a full range of 'cattle', which he introduced as the 'diseases of beastes'. First published in 1636, *The Countrymans Instructor* claimed to be based on 'my owne experience [of over thirty years] and the testimony of you my good friends', rather than on 'schollarship'.[38] Sixteen years later the work was republished in a slightly expanded version under the title of *The good-husbands jevvel*. This title continued to be use through multiple editions published through the end of the century, with the 1700 version rather oddly reiterating the claim that it was based on the author's experience over many decades.[39]

The most prolific English early modern writer about health care for horses was Gervase Markham. It has been suggested that his books targeted and were read by a 'thrifty, rural, middle class audience'.[40] Such a claim is supported by the promises Markham made in many of his books. *Markhams Methode, or Epitome*, for example, was said to provide remedies for 'all diseases whatsoever incident to Horses ... almost 300. All cured with twelve medicines only'. It also contained advice on how to rid cattle of diseases with seven medicines, sheep with six medicines and dogs with only three medicines.[41] These works continued to sell

---

[36] L. Mascal, *The husbandlye ordring and gouernmente of poultrie* (London, 1585), Sig. Aiiir and The *first booke of cattell* (London, 1591), sig A3v.

[37] M. Mendle, 'De Facto Freedom, De Facto Authority: Press and Parliament, 1640–43', *The Historical Journal*, 38, no 2 (June 1995), 307–332 and C. Webster, *The Great Instauration: Science, Medicine and Reform 1626–1660* (New York, 1976), p. 266.

[38] J. Crawshey, *The Countrymans Instructor* (London, 1636), sig. B1r and A2v.

[39] J. Crawshey, *The good-husbands jewel* (London, 1651 and London, 1700), sig. A1r.

[40] W. Wall, Renaissance National Husbandry: Gervase Markham and the Publication of England, *Sixteenth Century Journal*, 27, Vol 3 (1996), 767–85.

[41] G. Markham, *Markham's Faithfull Farrier* (London, 1638) and *Markhams Methode, or Epitome* (London: 1616), 30, 39 and 57.

long after his (unpublicised) death in 1637 and in the 1676 version of
one of his books, the introduction states that '[I] have now found out
the infallible way of curing all diseases in Cattle'.[42]

Although he alleged to have been a veterinary practitioner for fifty
years, his actual career was much more varied. As a young man,
Markham was a soldier in the Low Countries after which he held a
captaincy under Essex in Ireland. He appears to have been fluent in
Latin, French, Spanish, Italian and possibly Dutch. In 1616 he 'reviewed,
corrected, and augmented' the translation done by Richard Surflet of
Maison Rustique, or, the countrey farme by Chas Stevens and John
Liebault.[43]

There has been a great deal of debate over the years as to Markham's
actual qualifications for writing about animals. The author of *The Treatise of Horses*, John Lawrence, wrote in 1810 that Markham was 'nothing better than a mere vulgar and illiterate compiler'.[44] Lawrence's
comment, however, says more about Victorian attitudes than about the
period when Markham produced his works. As previously discussed,
gathering material from other sources and reproducing them in a 'new'
work was a common and accepted practice. *Markham's Master-piece
Revived*, included a list of the authors 'from whom any thing in this
Work is Collected, being the best Farriers':

> Xenophon, Rusticus, Vegetius, Pelagorious, Cameraius, Apollonius, Gres-
> son, Grilli, Horatio, Gloria de Caballi, Stevens, Wickerus, La Brove, Martin
> senior, Albiterio, Vinet, Clifford, Mascal, Markham. These are Private.
> Martin junior, Webb, Dallidown senior, Dallidown junior, Ashbourn,
> Stanley, Smith, Dowsing, Day, Barns, Mayfield, Lupan, Goodson, Parfray,
> White.[45]

Markham was also known to have copied from the work of the Thomas
Blundeville whose book *A new booke containing the arte of rydinge and
breakinge greate horses* was mentioned earlier in this chapter.[46] The tradition continued with writers such as Robert Almond, who confessed

---

[42] G. Markham, *A Way to Get Wealth* (London, 1661), sig. A1r.
[43] C.F. Mullett, 'Gervase Markham: Scientific Amateur', *ISIS*, Vol. 35, No 2 (Spring
1944) 106–118.
[44] J.F. Smithcors, *Evolution of the Veterinary Art: A Narrative Account to 1850*
(London, 1958), 193.
[45] G. Markham, *Markham's Master-piece Revived* (London, 1681), sig. A3r.
[46] R. Dunlop and D. Williams, *Veterinary History – An Illustrated History* (Chicago,
1996), p. 266.

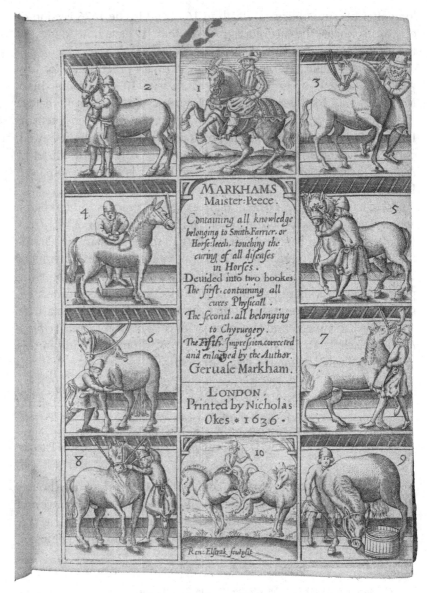

Fig. 4.1. Cover of G. Markham, *Markham's Maister-piece* (London, 1636).
Courtesy of the Wellcome Library, London.

that 'I owe much to my famous Countrey men Mr Blondevil, Mr Markham and Mr LeGrey, for that great light and knowledge'.[47]

Although compiling information from earlier works was regularly carried out, it was rigorously denounced by some writers. Thomas Grymes, for example, claimed that he only wrote about 'what is of my owne experience and practice, and whereof I have had good profile'. Thomas De Grey portrayed himself as a knowledgeable gentleman farmer who was interested in breeding horses. His book *The Compleat Horse-man and Expert Ferrier* claimed to offer 'a formall Examen of the office of the Ferrier'. A third writer condemned many popular books as being 'meere Collections out of others, and not their owne practice'. Ironically, all of these writers offered little more than a reworking of the material in Markham's books.[48]

Markham also wrote a number of books on health care for other 'beasts of burden' which were called *veterena* in Latin, which became the root of *veterinär* in German, or veterinary in English.[49] These included *Cheape and Good Husbandry* 'for the well-ordering of all Beasts and Fowles and for the generall Cure of their Diseases'. Other titles, which often appeared to be simply a different version of the same material, promised to contain advice on health care for all animals 'fit to the service of man'.[50]

Advice on animal health care could also be found in texts which combined human and animal medicine. Such works are often not easily identifiable by their titles, such as *The poor-mans physician and chyrurgion* or *The Dukes desk newly broken up: Wherein is discovered Divers Rare Receipts of Physick and Surgery* which appear to focus exclusively on humans.[51] There are also difficulties with trying to identify such texts through sources such as the *English Short Title Catalogue*. With over 460,000 items printed before 1801, this is a tremendously valuable

---

[47] R. Almond, *The English Horseman and Complete Farrier* (London, 1637), sig. A3r.

[48] T. Grymes, *The Honest and Plaine-deaing Farrier or a Present Remedy for curing Diseases and Hurts in Horses* (London, 1636), sig. A2r; T. De Grey, *The Compleat Horseman and Expert Farrier* (London, 1651), p. 61; R. Barrett, *The Perfect and Experienced Farrier* (London: 1660), sig. A2r and F. Smith, *Veterinary*, Vol 1 (note 13) 299, 303 and 321.

[49] A. Baranski, *Geschichte der Thierzucht und Thiermedicin* (Vienna, 1886), p. 17.

[50] Markham G.,*Cheape and Good Husbandry* (London: 1616), sig. A1r and *Way to Get Wealth* (note 27), sig. A1r.

[51] L. Coelson, *The poor-mans physician and chyrugion* (London, 1656) and W. Lovell, *The Dukes desk newly broken up: Wherein is discovered Divers Rare Receipts of Physick and Surgery* (London, 1661).

resource. However, since the catalogue only offers abbreviated titles and the fact that references to animals might only appear at the bottom of a title page, it is not always very useful for identifying books which combine human and animal medicine.[52]

Many texts which discussed both human and animal medicine were aimed at female readers, and included a mixture of food and medicinal recipes in addition to general household advice.[53] As the previous chapter explained, women were usually the first source of medical care for humans and tended to treat young or small animals, as well. *The Dukes Desk Newly Broken Up*, for example, offered 'rare receipts …good for all men, women and children together with several Medicines to prevent and cure most Pestilent Diseases in any Cattle'. *The Widdowes Treasure Plentifully Furnished with Sundry Secrets* included a number of remedies for horses, cows, bulls and 'steeres' alongside those for humans.[54]

'Herbals' or books on the nature and virtues of plants were also useful sources of information on the most common types of ingredients used in veterinary medicine. John Garard's *The herbal or Generall historie of plants* was first printed in Latin in 1596, but it appeared a year later in English and was reprinted regularly through the following century. It was followed by John Parkinson's herbal, the *Theatrum Botanicum* in 1640, Nicholas Culpeper's herbal in 1653 and Tay's herbal of 1686.[55] According to biographer Olav Thulesius, Culpeper's was the first herbal which actually 'set out to explain the virtues of his medicines and to deduce their action from astrological concepts'.[56] This seems a somewhat sweeping comment, although it is very true that Culpeper produced such comprehensive descriptions that editions of his herbal are still regularly reprinted for the use of modern practitioners of astrological medicine.

---

[52] British Library Online, http://estc.bl.uk [accessed October 2008].

[53] E. Tebeaux, 'Women and Technical Writing, 1475–1700' in L. Hunter and S. Hutton (eds.) *Women, Science and Medicine 1500–1700* (Stroud, 1997), pp. 33–40.

[54] J. Partridge, *The Widdowes Treasure Plentifully Furnished with Sundry Secrets: and Approved Secrets in Physicke and Chirurgery* (London, 1631), sig. F4r–6v; W. Lovell, *The Dukes Desk,* sig. A1r and C. Stevens and J. Liebault, *Maison Rustique, Or, The Countrey Farme,* (trans) Richard Surflet (London, 1616).

[55] J. Gerard, *The herbal or Generall historie. of plants* (London, 1597), sig. A2r; J. Gerard, *The herbal or Generall historie of plants,* ed. T. Johnson (London, 1633), sig. A2v and J. Parkinson, *Theatrum Botanicum: the Theatre of Plants or, an Herball of Large Extent* (London, 1640).

[56] O. Thulesius, *Nicholas Culpeper: English Physician and Astrologer* (London, 1992), p. 107.

As with all early modern herbals, these books not only contained descriptions of the various plants, but also provided advice on how to cultivate them, when to pick the plants and their medicinal uses for both humans and animals.[57] The large number of recipes found in early modern veterinary texts encompassed most common types of English garden herbs. Arsmart, or water pepper, for example, was said to have cooling and drying properties. This was considered to be a good restorative for horses; it was rubbed on their skin and with 'a good handful or two' of the herb also laid under the saddle. Savin was recommended for a variety of illnesses from killing worms in oxen, cows or calves to treating horses and sheep with unspecified complaints.[58]

Ephemeral Medical Literature

By 1500 there were printing presses in more than 250 European centre producing about twenty million copies for a population of less than eighty million resulting in what Peter Burke has called 'the commercialization of popular culture'. The term 'popular' has also been widely used in reference to 'literature' or 'the popular press'. It is not always clear what authors mean by this, although one commonly used definition is that of relatively cheap, small format books or other publications for non-specialists printed in a number of editions and sold in large numbers.[59] 'Popular' is also often used almost interchangeably with 'vernacular' which technically refers to texts written in the native tongue, in this case, English. In terms of medical literature, the word

---

[57] C.B. Atkinson and J.B., 'Anne Wheathill's A Handfull of Holesome (though Homelies) Hearbs (1584): The First English Gentlewoman's Prayer Book', *Sixteenth Century Journal*, 27 (Autumn, 1996), 659–672.

[58] N. Culpeper *Culpeper's Complete Herbal* (London, 1653), 16–17; J. Swan, *An Ephemeris* (Cambridge,1657), sig. C6r and W. Dade, *The Country-mans Kalendar* (London,1684), sig. B3r.

[59] P. Burke, *Popular Culture in Early Modern Europe*, second edition (Aldershot, 1994), p. 250; J. Barry, 'Literacy and Literature in Popular Culture: Reading and Writing in Historical Perspective' in T. Harris (ed.) *Popular Culture in England c.1500–1800* (London, 1995), p. 69; E.L. Furdell, *Publishing and Medicine in Early Modern England* (Rochester, 2002), p. 137; P. Isaac, 'Pills and Print' in R. Harris and M. Myers (eds) *Medicine, Mortality and the Book Trade* (1998), 25–49; L. Hunter, 'Books for daily life: household, husbandry, behaviour' in J. Barnard and D.F. McKenzie (ed.) *The Cambridge History of the Book*, IV (Cambridge, 2002), p. 515; and A. Johns, 'Science and the Book' in J. Barnard and D.F.M. McKenzie (eds) *The Cambridge History of the Book*, IV, 1557–1695 (Cambridge, 2002), 284.

'popular' can easily be confused with 'lay' medicine which implies a huge gap between university and non-university educated practitioners, which did not really exist.[60]

The second, although related problem, is the way in which medical literature has been identified and categorized. Lotte Hellinga has defined medical material produced before 1500 as that which 'serve[s] the physical well-being of mankind', including pharmacy, herbals, distillery and viniculture, alchemy, astrology, bloodletting, calendars and some almanacs. Paul Slack, on the other hand, uses a much narrower interpretation by suggesting that medical literature includes 'all books and pamphlets deliberately and largely devoted to the description, analysis or treatment of human health and disease.' This definition is honed still further by Ian Maclean who focuses on therapeutic and astrological topics.[61] While all three contain important elements, I would argue that there is a major problem with the fact that they omit texts on animal health care.

Popular veterinary literature could, however, be placed within either Hellinga's or Slack's definition. This encompasses a wide range of printed materials which discuss preventative and remedial veterinary medicine, aimed at consumers of various means and levels of literacy. The cheapest, and most accessible, were annual almanacs. Veterinary information was often found in agricultural texts on 'husbandry' in addition to works on the general care and breeding of animals. There were also many more easily identifiable as 'medical texts', some which covered both human and animal health and others which focused on the later.

There were many different types of medical literature available in early modern England. These ranged from erudite volumes in Latin and Greek aimed at a professional readership through 'popular' (ie written in the vernacular) books and pamphlets written for a broader audience. 'Ephemeral' literature includes many other categories such as broadsides, various forms of 'news-sheets' and almanacs. Although

---

[60] M. Pelling and F. White, *Medical Conflicts in Early Modern London: Patronage, Physicians, and Irregular Practitioners, 1550–1640* (Oxford, 2003), p. 10.

[61] L. Hellinga, 'Medical Incunabula' p. 76; P. Slack, 'Mirrors of health and treasures of poor men: the uses of the vernacular medical literature of Tudor England', in C. Webster (ed) *Health, Medicine and Mortality in the Sixteenth Century* (Cambridge, 1979), pp. 237–273 and I. Maclean, *Logic, Signs and Nature in the Renaissance: The Case of Learned Medicine* (Cambridge, 2002), pp. 40–41.

there are numbers of later seventeenth century newspapers in archives, the majority of ephemeral literature has not survived. As one author has duly noted, the 'fate' of most was 'to be recycled'.[62]

The genre of almanacs was a rare exception to this rule. There are fairly large numbers of surviving almanacs dating from the early sixteenth century. Printed and disseminated very year in December, the cheap, annual publications targeted, and were read by a wide cross-section of the public, making them the first true form of British mass media. Although their primary function was not to disseminate medical advice, most included some basic information. In general, this material focuses on 'popular' medicine, or traditional, Galenic principles and practices, with barely a nod to the great scientific discoveries of the seventeenth century, such as the circulation of blood within the body.[63]

Almanacs were amongst the first publications to be printed in the fifteenth century. Johannes Gutenberg published the first almanac in 1448, eight years before his famous Bible. By the 1470's large numbers of almanacs were being printed in various countries on the Continent and were particularly popular in Germany and the Netherlands.[64] Many of these almanacs were in a booklet form, while others appeared as broadsides, which were somewhat less in demand. Until the late sixteenth century, most printed English almanacs were translations of European ones which circulated along with English manuscript almanacs. The first almanac which was both written and produced in England is thought to be one by Andrew Boorde around 1537.[65]

Many writers provided material of interest to specific occupational groups ranging from weavers through to constables. *The City and Countrey Chapmans Almanack* included listings of markets and fairs, as well as mileage between towns and 'other things useful for all sorts of Traders'.[66] *The Sea-mans Almanack*, on the other hand, offered tide tables while *Veterinarium Meteorologist Astrology* provided a range of practical information on caring for livestock.[67]

---

[62] M. Mendle, 'Preserving the Ephemeral: Reading, Collecting and the Pamphlet Culture of Seventeenth Century England' in J. Andersen and E. Sauer (ed) *Books and Readers in Early modern England: Material Studies* (Philadelphia, 2002), 201–216.

[63] L. Hill Curth, *English almanacs*.

[64] R. Houston, *Literacy in Early Modern Europe* (London,1988), p. 180.

[65] B. Capp, *Astrology & the Popular Press: English Almanacs 1500–1800* (London, 1979), p. 27.

[66] *The City and Countrey Chapmans Almanack* (London, 1687), sig. A1r.

[67] *The Sea-mans Almanack* (London, 1655) and R. Gardner, *Veterinarium Meteorologist Astrology* (London, 1698).

Most surviving almanacs are made up of two major sections. The core of the first part always consists of a calendar marking upcoming astronomical and astrological events for the coming year. In most cases, this would be presented in a monthly format over two adjoining pages although some only contained one. This would include 'the Common aspects and configurations of the planets on a daily and/or weekly level.'[68] Depending on the size and format of the individual almanac, the calendars were often divided into two sections. On the left-hand side, every day was individually noted. Alongside these were listings for the time of 'the rising, southing and setting of the Planets.' These included the movements of the Moon, Saturn, Jupiter, Mars, Venus, Mercury and the Sun. On the right-hand side of the page, it was stand-ard form to include a space for miscellaneous information. In some cases, authors left part or all of this blank to use for personal notes. Surviving copies show that some people used this area to make notes about their business, the weather, health or current events.[69] The Oxford antiquarian Anthony Wood, for example, used both the supplied blank spaces in almanacs, as well as additional pages which he had bound in as a journal. Now held at the Bodleian Library in Oxford, his almanac-diaries contain notes on a range of topics, including numerous refer-ences to his business matters as well as events in Oxford such as several outbreaks of small-pox.[70]

The second section of almanacs was generally called the 'prognosti-cation'. This part usually contained material that was not as 'time-sensitive' as the astrological calculations in the first half. Depending on the author, these might include times and places of local markets, dis-tances between towns or medical information and advice. Joseph Blagrave, for example, offered the 'Time and Manner of curing Diseases by Sympathy and Antipathy, Rules for husbandry, dayly Predictions of the Weather, and many other Things beneficial for Phisitians and Young Students'.[71] Other provided details about therapeutic treatments,

---

[68] V. Wing, *An Almanac and Prognostication* (London, 1643), sig. A2r.

[69] See, for example, British Library Add. MS 4403, fl. 113-119b, Pell Papers, Diary in Samuel Morland's almanac, 1650;Add. MS 4956, William Courten (al. Charleton), Diary in Saunders' almanac, 1698; Add. MS 18,721; Sir Robert Markham, Bart. of Sedgebroke, Diary in Gadbury's almanac, 1681 and Buckinghamshire Records Office, D/X 581/2, John King of Steeple Claydon, Diary in Rider's *British Merlin*, 1687.

[70] T. Gallen, *An Almanack and Prognostication* (London, 1683), BODL, Wood Alm.b(6) and A. Wood, *Life and Times*, Vol. II, pp. 124, 133, 138 and 172.

[71] W. Blagrave, *Blagrave's Ephemeris* (London, 1659), sig. A1r.

recipes for medicines or preventative measures that could be taken to try to avoid becoming ill. In the latter part of the seventeenth century this might also include advertisements for proprietary medicines or medical services.[72]

Although the majority of health advice targets humans, many almanacs included information on preventative and remedial medicine for animals in this section. In some cases, this was fairly rudimentary advice. Two titles, however, targeted the occupational groups of shepherds and farriers. The *Calendarium pastoris or Shepherd's Almanack* was dedicated 'to the Shepherds and Plow-men of England' by John Bucknall. At first glance, this seems a surprising target audience, given the historical commonplace that labourers and men who took care of animals 'were for the most part illiterate'.[73] However, Bucknall specifically refers to himself as a shepherd who was inspired to study astrology and physick by the author and fellow shepherd 'Jo. Clearidge...in a little Book Printed in Anno 1670'. The stated purpose his first almanac in 1675 was so that his 'fellow Labourers' may receive 'the Fruit of what I have through hard study in the Wind and Wet obtained'.[74] Interestingly, Elizabeth Eisenstein's supposition that *The Shepherds Almanack* was probably read more by 'playwrights and poets then shepherds' suggests that she did not look at the text itself.[75] Unfortunately, actually proving that shepherds read this series is a more difficult proposition.

There are surviving copies of this series from 1675–1678 which suggests it was considered economically viable enough to run for more than one year. It is unclear whether it continued after this point or simply whether no copies have survived the centuries.[76] Despite the fact that Bucknall's almanac did not contain a great deal of veterinary advice, it did provide general information that a shepherd might need

---

[72] L. Hill Curth, *English Almanacs*, Chapter 9.

[73] J. Bucknall, *Calendarium Pastoris or The Shepherds Almanack* (London, 1675), sig. A1v; L. Wilkinson, *Animals and Disease: An introduction to the history of comparative medicine* (Cambridge: 1992), p. 10 and A. Wear, 'The Popularization of Medicine in Early Modern England' in R. Porter (ed.), *The Popularization of Medicine 1650–1850* (London, 1992), 17–34.

[74] See J. Claridge, *The shepheard's legacy* (London, 1670) and J. Bucknall, *Calendarium Pastoris or The Shepherds Almanack* (London, 1676), sig. A1v.

[75] J. Bucknall, *Shepherds Almanack* (1675), sig. A1v.

[76] For more information about almanac authors see L. Hill Curth, *English almanacs*, Chapter 3.

in his daily life. This included basic astrological tables about the movements of the planets and information such as how to 'finde the Moons Rising and Setting', the 'hour of the night by the Southing of the Stars' and how to make 'prognosticks by the Moon'. The main medical advice consisted of a remedy for sheep rot, the most serious disease that could afflict a flock. This was based on a mixture of powdered nutmeg and tar boiled in strong ale, which was to be fed to the affected animals 'two spoonfuls at a time, using it several times with two days distance between each time'.[77]

Veterinarium Meteorologist Astrology: or, the Farriers Almanacs, on the other hand, focused on the elite members of the domestic animal kingdom. Written by Robert Gardner who claimed to be a 'Student in Astrology and the compleat Art of Farrying', this almanac contained a range of recipes and other advice on remedial treatments. Although I have unable to study a surviving copy of his 1697 edition, his preface from the following year states that it had contained 'an Account of several Famous Medicines to prevent and cure many Diseases in Horses'. Furthermore, the title page of the sole surviving edition of 1698 title page promised to provide an 'account of several Famous medicines to Prevent and Cure many of the most Pestilential Diseases in Bullocks, Hogs, Sheep or any sort of Cattle' based on a combination of the wisdom of 'many good Authors and my own experience'. Gardner fulfilled this claim, by providing a range of generic recipes for 'cattle', as well as specific ones for bullocks, oxen, cows, lambs or hogs.[78] Unfortunately, while he also promised to provide an even more 'detailed discourse' about horses for the following year, it does not appear that any copies of this edition have survived.

Literacy and Readership

Many writers provided clues as to the types of audiences they were attempting to reach, either on the title page, in the preface to the reader or within the text itself. As previously mentioned, it does not necessarily follow that these were the people who actually purchased and/or read them. In fact, Elizabeth Eisenstein has suggested that title pages

---

[77] R. Gardner, *Veterinarium*, 1697, sig.A4v and C6r.
[78] R. Gardner, 1698, sig. A1r; A2r; A2v–7v.

provide only 'circumstantial evidence' as to their eventual circulation.[79] The same holds true for the men and/or women addressed in the preface of books, particularly if the work were dedicated to a member of the aristocracy or gentry. Similarly, a binding stamped with a royal coat of arms does not necessarily imply royal ownership, but could have meant that it was dedicated to the monarch.[80]

In her work on ephemeral literature printed twenty-five years ago, Margaret Spufford dramatically stated that the 'whole question of readership is maddeningly obscure'.[81] Other academics, however, believe that it is possible to draw at least some conclusions about early modern readers. Ian Maclean, for example, has argued that while 'until recently the reader was perhaps the most neglected element in the framework of literary communication' the tide had begun to change.[82] Over the past twenty years a number of academics working in a range of disciplines have addressed the topic of early modern readership from various angles. This has resulted in a variety of studies, some of which focus on specific literary genres, whilst others debate the 'politics' of reading.[83] However, none have solely addressed the readers of texts on the health and illness of animals.

In order to address these limitations this section will begin by addressing the key question of literacy or who would have been able to read texts on veterinary medicine. This will be followed by a discussion of the types of indirect evidence offered by the works themselves. Direct evidence of ownership or readership is, of course, more difficult to come by and it has been difficult to find inventories, library lists or wills

---

[79] E. Eisenstein, *The Printing Revolution in Early Modern Europe* (Cambridge, 1983), p. 34.

[80] D. Pearson, *Provenance Research in Book History: A Handbook* (London, 1994), p. 109.

[81] M. Spufford, *Small Books and Pleasant Histories: Popular Fiction and its Readership in Seventeenth Century England* (Cambridge, 1981), p. 258.

[82] I. Maclean, 'Reading and Interpretation' in A. Jefferson and D. Robey (eds) *Modern Literary Theory* (1986, 2nd edition), p. 122.

[83] See, for example, P. Slack, 'Mirrors of Health and Treasures of Poor Men: The Uses of the Vernacular Medical Literature of Tudor England' in C. Webster (ed.) *Health, Medicine and Mortality in the Sixteenth Century* (Cambridge, 1979), pp. 237–74; R. O'Day, *Education and Society 1500–1800: The Social Foundations of Education in Early Modern Britain* (London, 1982), pp. 193–4; A. Grafton, 'Studied for Action': How Gabriel Harvey Read his Library', *Past and Present*, 129 (1990), pp. 30–78; W.H. Sherman, *John Dee: The Politics of Reading and Writing in the English Renaissance* (Amherst, 1995) and A. Johns, *The Nature of the Book: Print and Knowledge in the Making* (Chicago, 1998).

that include such works. Hopefully, continuing research on the topic will uncover such proof in the future.

As previously mentioned, many of the early medical manuscripts were aimed at a 'professional' or 'educated' audience. With the advent of printing vast numbers of vernacular texts on animal health care became widely available to the general public. The first question to ask, therefore, is what kinds of people would have been able to read them? Until fairly recently, there has been a tendency to categorize people as either 'illiterate' or 'literate' with nothing in between. Today, this idea has fallen out of favour, for as Heidi Brayman Hackel has noted 'reading is a material and cognitive practice and changes over time and across culture'. In other words, our modern definition of what it means to be literate can not be directly applied to the early modern period.[84]

Before beginning a discussion on the types of people who were able to read vernacular medical books, one must begin with an explanation of what it means to 'read'. Kevin Sharpe has defined reading as a process 'in which we translate into our own words, symbols and mental contexts the marks and signs on the page'.[85] A prospective reader, therefore, would need to learn how to:

> know the letters within bookes and also the figures, and the numeracall letters...secondly to know and shew which are vowels, which consonants.[86]

Until fairly recently, the most popular method of determining literacy rested on the assumption that if a person were able to write their name, rather than simply leaving a mark, then they were also able to read. Adam Fox has suggested that the origins of this theory lay in the nineteenth century when elementary education was becoming widespread and a signature was used to signify literacy.[87] The continuing acceptance of this idea is illustrated in Lawrence Stone's theory of the 'hierarchy of literacy', first published in 1969. This defined the most elementary form of literacy as consisting of those who could 'read a little and sign

---

[84] H. Brayman Hackel, *Reading Material in Early Modern England: Print, Gender and Literacy* (Cambridge, 2005), p. 18.

[85] K. Sharpe, *Reading Revolutions: The Politics of Reading in Early Modern England* (New Haven, Conn., 2000), p. 34.

[86] T. Lambrocke, *Milke for children, or, A plain and easie method teaching to read and write* (London, 1685), p. 20.

[87] A. Fox, *Oral and Literate Culture in Early Modern England* (Oxford, 2000), p. 408.

their name'. The next level included the 'lower or middle classes with more reading, writing and use of numbers'. Stone's third level contained people who were educated enough to keep accounts and other business records. The fourth level included those who had sufficient education in the classics to go on to university. At the very top of the scale were men who either had gone to university and/or those who were members of an inn of court.[88]

Stones' theory has a number of flaws, the primary one being is that in the early modern period reading was taught before writing, and many students may never have progressed beyond learning to read. Furthermore, it suggests that literacy is a 'single, autonomous phenomena', when in fact, it can take many different forms at different times and although the ability to write almost certainly signifies the ability to read, the same does not hold true in reverse.[89] Finally, while learning to write fluently was a separate, secondary skill, producing a signature is a relatively easy thing to learn and does not necessarily mean that the person could produce anything else.[90] An individual might also have only have achieved a level of 'utilitarian' or functional literacy necessary for doing certain jobs, such as simple book-keeping. Recent studies have suggested that this was probably very common in social levels below the 'elite'. Joan Lane has argued that apprentices, for example, would have been required to be able to read and write. As discussed in the previous chapter, this would include young men who wished to become members of the Company of Farriers.[91] It seems likely that many other animal healers were also likely to need to keep at least form of rudimentary records.

---

[88] L. Stone, 'Literacy and Education in England 1640–1900', *Past and Present*, 42 (1969), p. 70.

[89] K. Thomas, 'The Meaning of Literacy in Early Modern England' in G. Baumann (ed) *The Written Word: Literacy in Transition* (Oxford, 1986), pp. 97–131.

[90] J. Simon, *Education and Society in Tudor England* (CUP, 1966), p. 376; B. Coward, *Social Change and Continuity in Early Modern England 1550–1750* (London, 1988), pp. 86–7; M. Spufford, 'First Steps in Literacy: The Reading and Writing Experiences of the Humblest Seventeenth-Century Autobiographers', *Social History*, 4, 3 (1979), pp 407–35 and D. Cressy, *Education in Tudor and Stuart England* (London, 1975), p. 75.

[91] A. Finkelstein, 'Gerard de Malynes and Edward Misselden: The Learned Library of the Seventeenth-Century Merchant', *Book History*, 3 (2000), 1–20; H.M. Jewell, *Education in Early modern England* (Basingstoke, 1998), p. 147–8; D. Simonton, 'Women and Education' in H. Barker and E. Chalus (eds) *Women's History: Britain, 1700–1850* (London, 2005), pp. 33–56 and J. Lane, *Apprenticeship in England 1600–1914* (London, 1996), p. 37.

There is a great deal of indirect evidence in title pages, prefaces and within the text, on what kinds of readers the various works were written for. Many appeared to have been targeting 'professional' and lay animal healers, or even owners. As the title *The Herds-man's mate* suggests, the book was aimed at those who 'take the charge or keeping this laborious, good, and fruitful kind of Cattle'.[92] Leonard Mascall's book on cattle, however, professed to be written both for 'the unlearned husbandman, as of the learned Gentlemen'.[93] A similar mixture of intended readers can be found in *The Gentleman's new jockey: or, Farrier's approved guide*, which promised to be 'of great Advantage not only to the Farmer, but even to the Professors and Practicers [sic] of these Arts too'.[94]

As previously mentioned, references to content or the target audience often only appear towards the end of a very long title. One such example is

> *The Modern Theory and Practice of Physic. Wherein The Antecedent Causes of Diseases; The Rise of the most Usual Symptoms incident to them; And the True Methods of Cure; Are Explained according to the Established Laws of Nature, and Those of the Animal Oeconomy.*[95]

There are, undoubtedly, a vast number of other early modern texts which have not yet been identified as containing veterinary-related content. It is hoped that further research on this topic will result both in the discovery of such work and in some form of definitive proof of the people who actually purchased and/or read these books.

Conclusion

Although texts on veterinary care go back to time immemorial, the advent of printing in the late fifteenth century dramatically transformed the way in which they were produced and distributed. The new technology swiftly spread throughout Europe and Britain, enabling the

---

[92] M. Harward, *The Herds-man's mate: Or, a guide for Herds-men* (Dublin, 1673), sig. A1r.

[93] L. Mascal, *The first booke of cattell* (London, 1587), Sig. A3v.

[94] G.L., *The Gentleman's new jockey: or, Farrier's approved guide* (London, 1691), p.154.

[95] B. Langrish, *The Modern Theory and Practice of Physic. Wherein The Antecedent Causes of Diseases; The Rise of the most Usual Symptoms incident to them; And the True Methods of Cure* (London, 1635).

reproduction of large numbers of identical images that could be widely disseminated to a local, regional or even national audience. As Lotte Hellinga has aptly noted, this allowed printers and publishers the opportunity 'to put at the disposal of a new class of readers the [medical] knowledge and experience accumulated over almost two millenia'.[96] The large number of medical titles and ephemeral literature such as almanacs produced in the early decades of mechanical printing suggests a great public interest in matters of health and illness. While many of these texts focused exclusively on humans, others jointly discussed human and animals, while a final category concentrated on animals.

The major theme of veterinary texts, from ancient manuscripts through early modern printed books, was that of continuity rather than change. Almost all of the advice on animal health care published in the early modern period was based on traditional, Galenic – humoural beliefs and practices. Writers appeared not to have been concerned with constantly offering new information or ideas, but rather on passing down the wisdom of earlier centuries. Many modern academics have negated the value of such compilations, arguing that it was little more than what we would now call plagiarism. This is nonsensical, as the value of their texts rested upon the perceived worth of the texts that they had been gathered from.

Ancient sources were seen as being highly reputable and most authors were proud to attribute their knowledge to ancient writers.[97] Such material appeared in a range of publications, including those which initially appear to focus exclusively on human health. It could also be found in husbandry or other agricultural works, as well as those that focused on the care of animals. There were also a number of almanacs which provided information about animal health care, albeit in a more rudimentary form than in clearly delineated 'medical' publications. Some actually referred to a target audience of shepherds, farriers or other types of agricultural workers, although there is no proof that such men were the actual consumers.

What is clear, however, is that there was a continuing demand for this type of literature. Many titles enjoyed a long life-span, appearing in numerous editions over time. In some cases, such as *The boke of*

---

[96] L. Hellinga, 'Medical Incunabula', p. 73.
[97] E. Gardiner, *Phisicall* [sic] *and approved Medicines* (London, 1611), sig. A3v and G. Markham, *Markham's Master-piece Revived* (London, 1681), sig. A3r.

husbandrie, they appeared under the name of a new author. Others, such as these texts originally written by Gervase Markham, were still attributed to him long after he had died. Almanacs, which were very small in size, could only carry a limited amount of information. Therefore, the continuing presence of medical advice in most almanacs suggests that this was something that consumers desired or even demanded.

Unfortunately, there appears to be little surviving proof of who purchased, owned or read veterinary texts. There are, however, a number of clues available within the texts themselves. The very long titles popular in this period often suggest what kinds of readers they were aimed at. Many writers also included prefaces which further expounded upon the type of people who would be interested in their work. As Gervase Markham reminded his readers,

> Thou shall finde in this [book] my Faithful Farrier, a Shoppe of Skil for thee to view. Let this bee thy Doctor, and they Druggist. Let this be thy Instructor and Director.[98]

---

[98] Ibid, *Markhams Faithfull Farrier* (London, 1638), sig. A3v-4r.

PART THREE

STRUCTURES OF PRACTICE

CHAPTER FIVE

'TO KEEP OUT DISEASE': PREVENTATIVE MEDICINE

> The art of Physicke by the judgment of the learned, hath two principall
> parts; the one declaring the order how health may be preserved: the other
> setting forth the meanes how sicknesse may bee remedies. Of these two
> parts (in mine opinion) that is more excellent, which preserveth health
> and preventeth sickness.[1]

'Medical models' help to explain the foundation and theory behind the
types of beliefs and practices that a society uses to deal with issues of
health and illness. Biomedicine, which is the dominant medical model
in Western Europe, focuses on disease rather than health. This is a relatively new concept, displacing the historical focus on both creating and
maintaining a state of health.[2] In the early modern period readers were
continually reminded that 'one of the most important businesses of this
Life, [was] to preserve our selves in Health'. This concept also applied to
trying to keep animals healthy, who were 'exceeding useful and service-
able to Man, and of no small value in themselves'.[3]

As discussed in Chapter 2, the concepts of what defines a state of
health differ according to the society and culture they take place in.
However, it seems likely that the early modern definition of animal
health was probably similar to that found in a recent survey of veterinary texts, as being the absence of disease.[4] There were thought to be
three basic types of phenomenon which would determine whether a
living creature was healthy or diseased. These consisted of 'thynges naturall', 'thynges not naturall' and 'thynges ageynst nature'. The first
included the unchangeable factors of four elements of earth, air, fire
and water which manifested themselves as the four humours. According
to Galenic thought, the second category of 'things non-natural' could

---

[1] T. Cogan, *The Haven of Health* (London, 1612), sig. A2r.

[2] L. Hill Curth, 'History of Health and Illness' in J. Naidoo and J. Wills (eds) *Health Studies: an introduction* (Basingstoke, 2008), pp. 47–68.

[3] P. Physiologus, *The Good housewife made a Doctor* (London, n.d.), sig. A2v, R. Saunders, 1681, sig. A7r. and W. Wadham, *England's Choice Cabinet of Rarities* (London, 1700), p. 3.

[4] S. Gunnarsson, 'The conceptualisation of health and disease in veterinary medicine', *Acta Veterinaria Scandinavica*, 2006, 48:20, 1–6.

alter one's humoral imbalance, whereby 'sicknesse is induced and the bodie dissolved' could be manipulated. These six non-naturals consisted of 'ayre', 'meate and drinke', 'slepe and watch', 'mevying and rest', 'empty-nesse and replettion' and 'affectations of the minde'.[5] The final category that could influence health consisted of 'contra-naturals', which literally meant against the naturals or 'thynges ageynst nature'. These consisted of pathological conditions made up of 'syckenesse, cause of syckenesse and accidents whiche foloweth syckenesse'.[6]

While little could be done to alter either the naturals or the contra-naturals, it was believed, in general, that the non-naturals could be manipulated. Since they were inter-related, the best way of doing this was by following a daily health regime based on living by 'Rule and wholesome Precepts'. Vegetius, writing in the fifth century, was the ear-liest author to stress the importance of good 'hygiene' for keeping ani-mals healthy. His advice included providing them with clean and warm housing where they could rest properly, well as ensuring that their food was neither 'musty or dirty'.[7]

Later medieval literature illustrates the continuing importance of providing domesticated, dependent animals with healthy housing and a good regimen. The thirteenth century writer Walter of Henley reminded readers that 'in order to exploit animals' labour, one has to care for them as well'.[8] As the previous chapter has illustrated, such advice became increasingly accessible after the advent of printing in the later part of the fifteenth century. These included texts such as *The Boke of Husbandrie* (1523) which stressed the importance of caring for one's animals. This included helping their animals maintain 'a good natural constitution, good digestion, good nourishment, moderation in feeding and diet, moderation in labour and sleeping and moderation in [sexual activities].[9]

---

[5] P.H. Niebyl, 'The Non-naturals', *British History of* Medicine, 45 (1971), pp. 486–492; T. Cogan, *The Haven of Health* (London, 1584), sig.A4r; L.J. Rather, 'The Six Things Non-Natural', *Clio Medica*, 3 (1968), pp. 337–347; S. Jarcho, "Galen's Six Non–Naturals," *Bulletin of the History of Medicine*, 44 (1970), pp. 372–377 and A. Boord, *A Compendious Regiment, or Dietarie of Health* (London, 1576), sig.A2r.

[6] T. Elyot, *The Castel of Health* (London, 1539), p. 1 and P. Gil Sotres, 'The Regimens of Health', in M.D. Grmek (ed) *Western Medical Thought*, pp. 291–318.

[7] E. Maynwaringe, *Vita sana & longa: the preservation of health and prolongation of life* (London, 1669), sig. A7v and F. Smith, *The Early History of Veterinary Literature* (London, 1912 and 1976), Vol I., pp. 24–5.

[8] J.E. Salisbury, *The Beast Within: Animals in the Middle Ages* (London, 1994), p 19.

[9] G.L. *The Gentleman's new jockey: or, Farrier's approved guide* (London, 1691), p. 42.

Although there has been a great deal of academic interest in 'healthy living' for humans in early modern England, little attention has been paid to the way in which the concept applied to animals.[10] There are a variety of possible reasons for this, beginning with prevailing anthropocentric views about medical history. On the other hand, it may be linked to the fact that it is much easier to identify texts on healthy lifestyles for humans because they generally contain 'regime' or 'regimen' in their titles. The earliest regimen manuals were written in Latin, but their increasing popularity meant that by the twelfth century a growing number were translated into Middle English or Anglo-Norman. With the advent of printing in the later part of the fifteenth century, the number of such works produced increased dramatically. There was some variation in these texts, with many concentrating most heavily on diet, while others covered the full range of the non-naturals. The sole unifying factor of regimen books, however, was that they focused exclusively on humans.[11]

The fact that a comparable literary tradition of such texts did not develop for animals does not mean, however, that such guidelines did not exist or that they were not disseminated to the general public. There is actually a great deal of information on early modern health regimens for animals, although it is somewhat more difficult and time-consuming to locate. Unlike manuals for humans, this advice is generally found scattered amongst the text of ephemeral literature such as almanacs, other medically oriented texts or more general works on agriculture and/or husbandry. Undoubtedly, much of this originated in the oral culture with evidence suggesting that much of it moved back and forth between the spoken word and print culture over time.

This chapter will piece together the advice and information provided in a variety of literary sources about how to keep ones animals healthy and disease free. The first section will examine contemporary ideas about 'healthy living' and illustrate how they applied to animals. As with

---

[10] See, for example, B.S. Turner, The Government of the Body: Medical Regimens and the Rationalization of the Body' *The British Journal of Sociology*, Vol 33, No 2 (June 1982), 254–269; P.G. Sotres, 'The Regimens of Health', pp. 291–319; L. Garcia-Ballester, 'Changes in the Regimina sanitatis: the Role of the Jewish Physicians in S. Campbell, B. Hall and D. Klausner (eds) *Health, Disease and Healing in Medieval Culture* (Basingstoke, 1992), 119–131.

[11] C. Rawcliffe, *Medicine & Society in Later Medieval England* (London, 1999), p. 37 and L.E. Voigts, 'Scientific and Medical Books' in J. Griffiths and D.A. Pearsall (eds.) *Book production and publishing in Britain 1375–1475* (Cambridge, 1989), pp. 345–402.

health regimes for humans, the basic principles were based on manipulating the Galenic non-naturals in order to prevent humoural imbalances. Therefore, the remainder of the chapter will discuss each of the non-naturals, the ways in which they could affect the health of animals and how they could be influenced.

Health Regimens

The concept of following a 'healthy lifestyle' is a familiar one to modern readers, who are constantly bombarded with messages from all forms of mass media. These range from advice on what to eat, how much to exercise or sleep to the importance of reducing excess stress in one's life. While many of these ideas claim to be based on 'modern' principles, most are almost identical to those propounded hundreds or even thousands of years ago.[12]

The earliest references date back to texts from the fifth century B.C. which discussed the important role diet played in maintaining a state of health. Hippocratic works such as *De prisca medicina* and *De diaeta* expanded the discussion to include other components of a healthy lifestyle. According to Pedro Gil Sotres, it was Galen's treatise *Hygieina* that marked the true starting point of what would eventually become an obsession with health and lifestyle. Some scholars might argue with his assertion that Galen exhibited a 'remarkable originality' or whether such ideas had been passed down from earlier generations. However, texts such as *Hygieina* made a definite contribution to ideas about how to have a healthy lifestyle and how this could change during the course of an individual's life.[13]

The evolution of these ideas can be seen in the number of medieval treatises on the subject, with the best known being the *Regimen sanitatis salernitannum* or *Salernitan Regime of Health*. Commonly credited to Arnald of Villanova (1240–1311), this was composed of verses which discussed the relationship between health and the Galenic non-naturals. The poem was associated with the tenth and eleventh century medical school of Salerno, a city which played a major role in the revival of classical medicine in the Christian West. Legend has it that its medical

---

[12] L. Hill Curth, 'Lessons from the past: preventative medicine in early modern England', *Journal of Medical Ethics: Medical Humanities*, 2003; 29, 16–21.

[13] P. Gil Sotres, 'Regimens', pp. 291–318.

school based its teachings on the writings of Hippocrates, said to have been brought to Salerno by a Latin, a Jew, an Arab and a Greek. Regardless of whether this was merely an apocryphal story, it was presumably meant to suggest that the regimen was universally supported by members of the medical profession. In any case, the *Salernitan Regime of Health* became so popular that it appeared in at least 240 versions in Latin and multiple editions in English and other European languages over the following centuries. It seems likely that the format of the text made it simple for people skilled in mnemonic powers to memorize its basic principles.[14]

It has long been a historical commonplace that the readership of such manuals was restricted to the social elite or the middle and upper sections of society for much of the late medieval and early years of the Renaissance. In 1979, for example, Paul Slack argued that only a 'certain class' would have read these books and acted upon them. More recent works have suggested that the regimens of health were particularly attractive to physicians who could use them to design a course for his patients.[15] Ken Albala, however, believes that there were three separate phases in the development of regimen books and correspondingly different audiences. He agrees that courtiers and other members of elite society were the main consumers of these works from roughly 1470–1530. However, Albala feels that the following period of 1530–1570 was a time of transition to a new form of literature that targeted a broader audience. His third and final period runs from the 1570's into the 1650's with a range of new writers, many of whom attempted to modernise the classical advice that had been the basis of previous works. It was also a period of dramatic growth in ephemeral literature with a correspondingly wide target audience. These views are supported by the material on health regimens in found in contemporary almanacs, the first true form of British mass media that were introduced in Chapter 3.[16]

---

[14] R. Porter, *The Greatest Benefit to Mankind*, (London, 1997), p. 107 and A. Fox, *Oral and Literate Culture in England 1500–1700* (Oxford, 2000).

[15] P. Slack, 'Mirrors of Health', 237–74; C. Rawcliffe, *Medicine and Society*, p. 37 and R. French, *Medicine before Science: The Business of Medicine from the Middle Ages to the Enlightenment* (Cambridge, 2003), p. 120.

[16] K. Albala, *Eating Right in the Renaissance* (Berekley, California, 2002), pp. 26–37 and L. Hill Curth, *Almanacs, astrology and popular medicine, 1550–1700* (Manchester, 2007).

Interestingly, all of the modern academic discussions about health regimens have been limited to literature about humans. As previously stated, this may be partially explained by the absence of a parallel genre of 'regimen' books for animals. It can not, however, be justified by the paucity of comparable texts on healthy lifestyles for animals. On the contrary, there were copious amounts of printed information on how to provide domesticated animals with a healthy lifestyle. Unlike texts for humans, however, these works did not contain the words 'regime' or 'regimen' in their titles. Instead, this material was generally combined with other types of useful information on animal care. Depending on the author, this might include advice on buying, feeding and breeding animals through to more comprehensive texts that covered most aspects of an agricultural lifestyle. Given the importance allocated to preserving a state of health, it is hardly surprising to find that many texts discussed both the role that a healthy lifestyle played in preventative medicine, alongside therapeutic methods.

Animals and the Six Non-naturals

> The Six which are not Natural be the Air, Meat and Drink, Motion and Reset, Sleep and Watch, Emptiness and Fullness and the Affects or Motions of the Mind: and these are called not natural, because as (being rightly and in due order applied) they preserve sustain and fortifie the Body; so being most governed or sed in any excess or disorder, they are the only corrupt Destroyers of the whole body.[17]

Ayre [Air]

> The ayre cannot be too cleane and pure considering it doth close, and doth compasse us round aboute, and we doe receive it into us, we cannot be without it for we live by it…[18]

It is hardly surprising that the first non-natural focused on the all encompassing element of air. The ancient Greeks believed that air was 'the most powerful of all things', linked not only to human and animal life, but also to the transmission of disease. In the early modern period, there were a range of gradients for what constituted 'good' or 'bad' air

---

[17] G. Markham, *Markham's Master-piece Revived* (London, 1681), p. 1.
[18] A. Boorde, *A Compendious Regiment, or Dietarie of Health* (London, 1576), sig. A6v.

with the aim being to try to 'Keepe your selfe in a pure Ayre'.[19] However, it must be remembered that the definition of 'clean' air is a function of early modern society and culture, and might not have been the same in the sixteenth as in the twenty-first century one. For example, what is now referred to as 'air pollution' is said to emanate from a number of sources, including industry, agriculture, services, households, solid waste management, and road, air, and sea transport.[20] With the exception of air transport, all of these factors also featured in the creation of early modern miasma, joined by 'emanations from the earth' and 'the perspirations of vegetable and animal substances'. The former involved noxious vapours caused by subterranean heat which would rise up and contaminate the air, while the later would ferment, putrefy and sink into the soil, only to be spewed back at a later time.[21] As a result, areas such as battlefields, which combined both vapours from the soil and from decomposing bodies, were widely perceived to have unhealthy air. The combination of these fumes with the exhaust of gunpowder was particularly dangerous both to soldiers and their animals, as well as those living in surrounding areas. If the site then become waterlogged, as well, the potential for disease became even greater. As one writer reminded readers, 'Gros Air or evil Scents' would not only make an animal 'loath his Provender but corrupt the Blood and subject the whole body to Diseases'.[22]

It was thought that the air quality differed dramatically in far-flung parts of the world, with the air in one's place of birth being healthier than in other locations. Unlike regimen books, which often went into great detail about air quality, works addressing animal health generally did not. This may have been due to a lack of space in more general medical or agricultural works compared to manuals on a regimen salutis. Secondly, as with humans, many animals would be born and die in the same general areas while others might travel (or be transported) to faraway lands. Therefore, the majority of working animals would

---

[19] C.R.S. Harris, *The Heart and the Vascular System in Ancient Greek Medicine: from Alcmaeon to Galen* (Oxford, 1973), p. 43; J. Longrigg, *Greek Rational Medicine: Philosophy and medicine from Alcmaeon to the Alexandrians* (London, 1993), pp. 76–78; V. Nutton, 'The Seeds of Disease' in *From Democedes to Harvey* (London, 1988), XI, pp. 1–34 and T. Langley (London, 1643), sig. B3r.

[20] L. Hill Curth, 'Lessons from the past', pp. 16–20.

[21] A. Corbain, *The Foul & The Fragrant: Odour and the Social Imagination* (London, 1996), pp. 13 and 22–3.

[22] C. Carlton, *Going to the Wars: The Experience of the British Civil Wars, 1638–1651* (London, 1996), p. 223 and G.L. *Gentleman's new jockey*, p. 49.

probably have spent their lives in roughly the same area, and air, in which they were born.

It is true, however, that some animals may have moved often great distances during their lifetimes. These would have included certain types of animals, such as cattle and sheep, who were transported to urban centres such as London to provide fresh meat. Since the beginning of the sixteenth century, for example, Welsh cattle were regularly driven to England for slaughter. Of course, it seems unlikely that there would have been much concern about the health of animals that would shortly be slaughtered.[23]

Horses, however, were a much more valuable commodity and would have been a matter of greater concern. This probably holds especially true with the importation of extremely expensive foreign horses during the course of the later seventeenth and eighteenth centuries. The first Arabian horses were imported into England during the reign of James I, followed by a rapidly accelerating number of various other types of 'oriental' animals.[24] Although many of the non-naturals could be manipulated to try to keep them healthy, little could be done about the 'foreign' air in their new homes.

Although the air was best in one's birthplace, there were many gradients of 'good air' in other places. On the broadest level, this could be linked to the sign of the Zodiac linked to the country and more specifically to the town or area in question. England, for example, fell under Aries and was therefore linked to Mars. In theory, this meant that those born in this country would share some general physical and behavioural characteristics. The former would include 'a dry body of middle stature, lean and spare, big bones [and] strong thick shoulders'. This would be altered further by the town in which one was born. London, for example, was linked to Gemini which shared the humoural characteristic of heat with Aries, but which was moist rather than dry. York, on the other hand, was linked to the cold and moist sign of Cancer. Interestingly, cities such as Constantinople and Tunis also fell under the sign of Cancer. This suggests that a horse imported from that part of the world was likely to find the air healthier in the north of England, than in the south.[25]

---

[23] M. Overton, *Agricultural Revolution in England: The transformation of the agrarian economy 1500–1850* (Cambridge, 1996), p. 139.

[24] P. Edwards, *Horse and Man in Early Modern England* (London, 2007), pp. 110–11 and R. Dunlop and D. Williams, *Veterinary Medicine: An Illustrated History* (Chicago, 1996), pp. 237 and 480.

[25] W. Eland, *A Tutor to Astrology. Or, Astrology made easie.* (London, 1694), pp. 4–5 and 19–20.

In practical terms, the air in rural areas was thought to be cleaner than in densely populated towns.[26] However, while little could be done to alter the general characteristics of the air in the place where one lived, it was possible to improve the quality within animal shelters. Cleanliness was the key-note, even for 'the most filthy....swine'. At the very least, this meant keeping their housing well ventilated, dry and warm, in order to prevent animals from becoming chilled. 'Low, wide houses like Barns' or 'low, long and broad' buildings were often recommended as being easier to 'be warm in the winter', when even the hardiest animals would need some shelter from the elements.[27]

Air temperature, particularly the 'intemperature of the Aire' was also considered to be a major factor in the spread of disease.[28] Animals which were cold and moist by nature, such as sheep, would be at particular risk during the winter and during an unseasonable spring. Large amounts of rain, which resulted in 'floated Ground or boggy land' was thought to be the harbinger of sheep rot. In order to protect their health, shepherds were advised to provide them with dry shelter rather than to 'work them ... a time too cold or too wet'. However, all types of animals could be affected by air fouled by misty or foggy weather, particularly after sunset.[29]

Windy weather also helped spread diseases which could be carried and transmitted over great distances through 'ill ayre'. These included highly contagious illnesses such as small pox and measles, as well as malarial fevers and intestinal infections which could even turn into a plague epidemic.[30] The direction of the winds was also thought to have a major impact on health. Gusts from the east were thought to be cold and could result in 'sharp feavers, raging madnesse, and perilous Aposthumations', while those from the south were hot and moist and 'breedeth corrupt humours and in hot bodies cramps, giddinesse in the head,

---

[26] A. Wear, 'Making Sense of Health and the Environment in Early Modern England' in *Medicine in Society: Historical Essays* (Cambridge, 1992), pp. 120–43.

[27] F.B., *The Office of the Good Housewife* (London, 1672), p. 31; W. Lovell, *The Dukes desk newly broken up: Wherein is discovered Divers Rare Recipts of Physick and Surgery*, (London, 1661), p. 9; T. Tryon, *The country-man's companion: or, A New Method of Ordering Horses & Sheep So as to preserve them both from diseases and casualties* (London, 1688), pp. 12–13; ibid., *The Way to Save Wealth; Shewing how a Many may Live plentifully for Two-pence a day* (London, 1695), p. 45 and A.S., *The husbandman, Farmer, and Grasier's Compleat Instructor* (London, 1697), p. 59.

[28] M. Harward, *The Herds-man's Mate*, p. 1.

[29] J. Claridge, *The Shepheard's Legacy* (London, 1670), p. 27 and Anon, *A Help to Discourse, or More Merriment mixt with Serious Matter* (London, 1682), p. 165.

[30] A. Boorde, *A Compendious Regiment, or Dietarie of Health* (London, 1576), sig. A6v.

or the falling sicknesse, pestilence and cruel fevers.'[31] Unlike humans, however, animals spent the majority of their time in the open air. However, the forecast of particularly dangerous winds could be met by minimizing the time they spent outside their housing.

Meat and Drink

> Diet is as important for animals as for humans for prevention of illness...[32]

Dietetics has been called one of the most ancient branches of the therapeutic art, despite the fact that our modern definition is somewhat different than it was in the past. In the early modern period 'dietetics' encompassed a range of considerations, from the humoural qualities of different types of food and drink to the most appropriate times for consumption.[33] The Hippocratic text *On Ancient Medicine* suggests that 'in the beginning' both humans and beasts were able to be 'nourished, grow, and lead their lives free of trouble' by eating 'fruits, brush, and grass'. It goes on to say that while such a 'strong and brutish regimen' continued to suit animals, humans were forced to 'seek forms of more differentiated forms of nourishment better suited to their constitutions.'[34] The types of food and drink that this referred to did, of course, change dramatically over the centuries in response to social, cultural and economic factors.

Galen's three-book 'On the Powers of Food', written about 180 A.D, classified all foods according to their individual properties. As Galen pointed out, every type of living creature had a unique balance, which changed during the course of the life cycle, and which needed to be identified and catered for. Since most domesticated animals were unable to source their own food, it was up to the owners to make sure that they did not 'endanger the health' of their charges. According to one author, 'moderation in eating is another main cause of Long Life, as immoderate Eating is of a short one.'[35] Humans were, therefore, expected

---

[31] N. Culpeper, *Galen's Art of Physick* (London, 1657), p. 123 and Swallow, 1699, sig. B5v.

[32] G. Markham, *A Way to Get Wealth* (London, 1676), p. 40.

[33] J. O'Hara-May, 'Food or Medicines? A Study in the Relationship Between Foodstuffs and Materia Medica Sixteenth to Nineteenth Centuries', *Transactions of the British Society for the History of Pharmacy*, I (1971), p. 63.

[34] Hippocrates, *On Ancient Medicine*, (trans) M.J. Schiefsky (Leiden, 2005), p. 77.

[35] J. Wiseman, *The Pig: A British History* (London, 2000), p. 77: J. Mortimer, *The whole art of husbandry: or, the way of managing and improving of land*. (London, 1721), p. 249: M. Grant, *Galen on Food* pp. 68–190 and V. Nutton, *Ancient Medicine* (London, 2004), pp. 240–241.

to monitor both the consumption of animals being fed at home or in pastures. According to one seventeenth-century author, cattle were so greedy that they liable to 'eat themselves sick' if let for too long in a field full of sweet, tasty clover.[36] This view continued into the following century with some writers arguing that the over-consumption of rich or 'unwholesome' herbs was a major factor in reoccurring bouts of 'cattle plague'.[37]

In general, advice on what to feed animals changed relatively little during the early modern period. The major exceptions were due to changes in agricultural and distribution systems. By the mid-seventeenth century, such methods had already reached the point where English society could escape 'wholesale, repeated famines'. In fact, 1650–1770 is often referred to as 'the period of great agricultural development' with an almost continuous introduction of new crops and work on rotating crops.[38] As the final chapter will discuss, there were a number of 'agricultural societies' formed in the eighteenth century to discuss such issues. The Odiham Society, which played a role in the foundation of the first London Veterinary College in 1792, also offered premiums to promote good ploughing, distributed seeds for controlled experiments and arranged for demonstration of farm machinery.[39]

The cost of growing sufficient crops to feed animals could be very high. At Tydal in the 1690's, for example, the agistment charge for keeping an ox on Fleming's demense lands was normally 6 pence per week. Since the price of beef during the period was approximately 3 pence per pound, Fleming's oxen needed to put on at least 2 pounds every week to even meet the costs of their feed. Winter stall-feeding of a bullock to bring it to prime condition required a ration of at least two hundred weight of hay a week for up to twenty weeks. An alternative method of cold-weather care consisted of keeping sheep in the house, and feeding them a mixture of beans, ground round, bran, and

---

[36] R. Blome, *The gentlemans recreation in two parts* (London, 1686), p. 50.

[37] J. Smith, *Profit and pleasure united: or, the husbandman's magazine* (London, 1704), p. 85; T. Bates, 'A brief account of the contagious disease which raged among the milch cowes near London, in the year 1714', *Philosophical Transactions*, 1718, 30: 872–885, p. 884 and *London Magazine, or, Gentleman's Monthly Intelligencer*, 1745, p. 598.

[38] E.L. Jones, *Seasons and Prices: The Role of the Weather in English Agricultural History* (London, 1964), p. 54; C. Shammas, *The Pre-Industrial Consumer in England and America* (Oxford, 1990), p. 121 and J. Lerner, 'Science and Agricultural Progress: Quantitative Evidence from England, 1660–1780', *Agricultural History*, Vol 66, 4 (Autumn, 1992), pp. 13–14.

[39] P. Horn, 'The Contribution of the Propagandist to Eighteenth-Century Agricultural Improvement', *The Historical Journal*, Vol. 25, No. 2 (Jun., 1982), pp. 313–329.

a few oats. By the latter part of the century new food crops such as clover and turnips provided enough nourishment to over-winter larger numbers of animals successfully. The latter became popular for feeding animals in the second half of seventeenth century. In 1659 one author recommending fattening hogs and horses 'in a trice' with 'Turnip-bread' which was 'a new and late devise' [sic]. However, most authors suggested including turnips as part of a time-honoured diet of oats and other grains which might be mixed with some 'Beanes or Pease, well dried and hard'. In the case of pigs, this might have produced better tasting meat, for although turnips were good to 'fatten them very much' too many could result in the animal having the 'tast [sic] of the turnup'.⁴⁰

The types of foods that were fed to animals differed according to their humoural qualities, as well. Horses, for example, were considered to be predominantly hot and dry animals, as were 'swine'. It therefore benefited both to have 'cold Herbs, or Lettice, Endive, Succory, Violet leaves, Dandelion [and] Sow thistle' mixed into their feed during the summer to keep them from falling ill. In other words, a good preventative diet would include foods that were cooling and moistening. Sheep, on the other hand, were better off feeding 'upon the salt and short pasture' which would ensure that they would 'live in health'.⁴¹

Sleep and Watch

> Concerning the quantity or time how long wee should sleep, it cannot bee certainly alike defined for all men…It must be measured by health and sicknesse, by age, by emptinesse or fullnesse of the body & by the complexion.⁴²

Sleep was an important component of the Galenic health regime, and much discussed in early modern medical works on human health care. There were various beliefs related to sleep, based on the idea that it

---

⁴⁰ J. Thirsk, *The Agrarian History of England and Wales*, Vol. II (Cambridge, 1985), p. 104; T.E. Gibson, *A Cavalier's Note Book* (London, 1880), pp. 187–8; E. Gayton, *The art of longevity, or, A diaeteticall institution* (1659), p. 14; G.. Markham, *Cheape and Good Husbandry* (1614), p. 3; and J. Percival, *The English Travels of Sir John Percival and William Byrd II*, (ed) M.R. Wagner (Columbia, Missouri, 1989), p. 54.

⁴¹ T. Tryon, *The country-man's companion*. p 2; J. Blagrave, The Epitome of the Art of Husbandry (London, 1670), p. 127 and E. Toppsell, *The Historie of Foure-Footed Beastes* (London, 1607), p. 467.

⁴² T. Venner, *Via recta ad vitam longam, or, A plain philosophicall demonstration* (London, 1638), p. 279.

allowed the innate heat of the body to be returned to the internal organs, which in turn would aid digestion and help the body to repair itself. According to Nicholas Culpeper, the time spent sleeping would 'comfort nature much, refresheth the memory, cheers the spirits, quickens the senses'. The same held true for animals, for whom sleep had been 'ordained by Nature to ingender strength'.[43]

The correct amount of sleep for an animal depended on a range of factors. Firstly, it would be linked to the kind and amount of work that they were doing. Secondly, these needs were likely to change as they aged during the course of their lives. Horses, for example, were thought to require more, as well as to sleep better when they were older.[44] Dogs were said to 'sleep as doth a man, and therein dream very often, as may appear by their often barking in their sleep'. However, the author noted that, as with humans, they should not be allowed to sleep immediately after eating.[45]

That said, as with the other non-naturals, moderation was the key word for sleeping habits for 'Long and superfluous Sleep' could 'chill the Body, weaken the Natural Heat and breed Flegmatic Humours.' As one author reminded readers, while 'too much waking is an Enemy to Health...excessive sleeping dozes the Brains, hinders digestion and obstructs Nature in the Performance of her Offices'. Gervase Markham believed that animals who slept 'unto excess' were either suffering from lethargy or had 'some inward grief'. Sick animals might also appear 'dull and sleepy', a sign also apparent in humans who were 'oppressed with sleep, and are sluggish and idle'.[46]

Labour, Rest and Exercise

> If he [man] eats or drinks plentifully in a Morning and then presently labour strongly, or go a Journey after it, unless he be very moderate therin,

[43] K.H. Dannenfeldt, 'Sleep: Theory and Practice in the Late Renaissance', *The Journal of the History of Medicine and Allied Sciences*, 41 (1996), p. 415; G.P. Sotres, 'Heath Regimens', p. 310; N. Culpeper, *Galen's Art of Physick* (London, 1657), p. 129; G. Markham, *Markham's Master-piece Revived* (London, 1681), p. 14 and G.L., *The Gentleman's new jockey* , p. 49.

[44] S. Solleysel, *The Parfait Mareschal or complet Farrier*, (trans) Sir W. Hope (Edinburgh, 1696), p. 17.

[45] E. Toppsell, *Four Footed Beastes*, p. 110.

[46] G. Markham, *Maister-piece*, p. 13; L. Laevinus, *The Secret Miracles of Nature* (London, 1658), p. 122 and T. Watson, *Instructions for the Management of Horses and Dogs* (London, 1785), p. 47.

he shall find himself much indisposed the first part of the day…the very same is to be understood in other Creatures[47]

The need to consider the relationship between 'labour' and 'rest' was as important for working animals as it was for humans. Although these included moral considerations, in the case of animals the primary motivation was probably economic. The consequences of over-work might cause a 'weakness or poorness of body' or might eventually result in 'some disease or the other' including the potentially fatal 'pestilence', all of which would result in a non-productive beast.[48] On more moral lines, many believed that all animals were entitled to a weekly day of rest. However, although little could be done to stop individual farmers from working their animals on a Sunday at home, an Act of 1628 forbade drovers, carriers and waggoners from travelling anywhere on the Sabbath.[49]

Since animals carried out many different types of work, the balance between work and rest would have varied widely. Horses living on a farm might be expected to help prepare the ground for planting, pull ploughs or other machinery as well as the carts or wagons which took goods to market. They were also used to carry people in commercial or private vehicles such as coaches, as well as for a variety of tasks during warfare.[50] In addition, horses and many other types of animals were used in sporting, recreational or other potentially tiring activities. The reoccurring outbreaks of war in the early modern period also meant that many horses would serve on battlefields, where it might be difficult to find a safe place for rest.

The central unifying factor was that both labour and rest were to taken in moderation. Gervase Markham said that horses needed to be set 'fit times and seasons for sleeping and waking'.[51] It was suggested that horses exhausted by 'hard labour' or 'over-riding' should be 'well rubbed' then allowed to rest for up to three hours. Racing horses, on the other hand, were expected to conserve their strength and only be allowed to

---

[47] T. Tryon, *The country-man's companion*, p. 6.

[48] W. Dade, *An Almanack* (London, 1684), sig. B3r and L. Mascal, *The Government of Cattle* (London, 1662), p. 6.

[49] G. Cross, *A Social History of Leisure Since 1600* (State College, PA, 1990), p. 29 and M. Reed, *The Making of Britain: The Age of Exuberance 1550–1700* (London, 1986), p. 244.

[50] See P. Edwards, *Horse and Man* for a detailed description of the various roles horses played in early modern England.

[51] G. Markham, *The Complete jockey* (London, 1695),

run two 'matches' a week. In addition, it should be allowed to sleep from nine in the evening until 'just before sunrise' the next day.[52]

A dog which was used for strenuous jobs such as hunting or 'fowleling', either on land or water would have required a proportionate amount of time to recuperate. Herding would also have been a tiring job, particularly when 'exercising' sheep, a task which consisted of chasing them 'up and down till they are weary'. Since both dog and sheep would have been weary afterwards, it was suggested that this be followed by a period of rest for all involved. John Caius' classic *Of Englishe Dogges* lists a number of dogs which also had very draining jobs. These included the 'Daunser ... which are taught and exercised to daunce in measure at the musicall sounde of an instrument' and the 'Turnespete' who worked hard to keep the joint of meat turning on a spit over the fire. Pet dogs, on the other hand, were likely to need less rest. These included 'delicate, neate and pretty kind of dogges' such as 'the Spaniel gentle, or the comforter' who spent their days being played or 'dallied' with by their female owners.[53]

Emptinesse and Repletion

> Physicks that evacuate are divers, for some do sensibly evacuate the Matter by the Belly, by Vomits, by Urine, by Sweat, by Spittle, by the Palate, by the Nostrils.[54]

The belief that good health was linked to the periodical removal of excessive humours meant that purging was regularly carried out as a preventative measure, as well as to cure diseases.[55] The modern definition of purging generally refers to the emptying of the bowels or stomach. However, in early modern England century this was only one of many different methods used to remove various unwanted materials from the body. Others included vomiting or 'neesing' [sneezing] and using 'clysters' [enemas] or diuretics. Phlebotomy, depending on where the blood was let from, could purge all sections of the body. 'Sweating',

---

[52] T. Tryon, *Country-man's Companion*, p. 7 and R. Almond, *The English horsman and complete farrier* (London, 1671), pp. 31–3.

[53] J. Caius, *Of Englishe Dogges* (London, 1576), pp. 4, 14, 20 and Anon., *A treatise of oxen, sheep, hogs and dogs with their natures, qualtities and uses* (London, 1683), pp. 35 and 22.

[54] N. Culpeper, *Medicaments for the Poor or Physick For the Common People* (London, 1670), p. 2.

[55] J. Booker, *Telescopium Uranicum* (London, 1661), sig. A8r and F. Beridge, *Ephemeris* (London, 1654), sig. B3r.

on the other hand, was a more general method of cleaning unwanted substances from the system.

Almost all of the procedures that were used for humans were also applied to animals. The few that were not would have been because of the difficulty in carrying out the procedures. It seems unlikely, for example that 'gargarismes' or gargles could be administered to an animal. There were also some differences in the types of ingredients used. As the following chapter will show, while all were based on herbal, or other organic items, those for animals were generally called for cheaper and more easily accessible products.

One of the most frequently recommended methods of purging for preventative reasons was, phlebotomy, which comes from the Greek words 'phleps' or vein, and 'tome' or incision, was. Many writers recommended the periodical or regular letting of blood in order to 'prevent disease and so preserve health'.[56] That said, there was a great deal of debate as to how and when this should be done. Unlike bloodletting for acute illnesses, there was more flexibility as to when preventative phlebotomy could be carried out. In general, this was to be done either in the spring or fall when the weather was still temperate. Theoretically, the blood was to be let from the right side during the former and from the left in the fall or winter.[57] William Dade recommended making an incision on the neck of horses, and drawing blood on the first day of April to make them stay healthy 'the whole year'. Some other writers agreed with this, while many more recommended the procedure be done either every quarter or twice a year.[58]

The actual timing for the procedure depended on the phases of the moon, some of which threatened danger, or even death. This was based on the idea that the amount of blood in the body ebbed and flowed in response to its movements. As a result, it was dangerous let blood 'within three dayes before or after the Change of the Moone' because the procedure might cause the animal to bleed to death. It was also important

---

[56] T.E. Crowl, 'Bloodletting in Veterinary Medicine', *Veterinary Heritage*, 1 (1996), p. 15; R. Almond, *The English Horsman and Complete Farrier* (London, 1637), p. 57; H. Rogeford, *An Almanack* (London, 1561), sig. D2r and J. Evans, *Almanack* (London, 1629), sig. B8r.

[57] E. Voigts and M.R. McVaugh, A Latin Technical Phlebotomy and Its Middle English Translation in Transactions of the American Philosophical Society, New Ser., Vol 74, 2 (1984) 1–69.

[58] W. Dade, *The Country-mans Kalendar* (London, 1700), sig. B4v; G. Markham, *Cheape and good* husbandry, p. 46 and L.W.C., *The English Farrier, Or, Country-mans treasure* (London, 1639), sig. A4r.

to avoid letting blood 'within 24 houres before nor after the full' because this was when the humours would be in the process from flowing from the interior to the exterior of the body. Finally, it was vital to know when the Moon was in aspect with Jupiter, 'the giver of life' as this which could also result in the loss of excessive amounts of blood.[59]

Affectations of the Mind

> The passions, motions or perturbations of the minde, which otherwise may be called the accidents of the spirit, are strange or sodaine insurections and rebellious alterations of a tumultuous troubled soule.[60]

As previously discussed, early modern medicine was based on the holistic model which 'presumed unity of body and behaviour with the physical and the psychological two sides of the same coin'.[61] The final of the non-naturals best illustrates this relationship by emphasising the link between feelings and emotions and physical health. There were various medical explanations as to how an excess of passions would lead to illness. One theory was that giving free reign to any of them would 'divert the vital heat from the circumference to the centre'. This would result in the body being weakened which could result in a range of mental or physical disorders. Wrath, for example, could produce such an intense level of heat that it could result in 'frenzy'. Sloth or excessive disappointment, on the other hand, could generate a corresponding level of coldness.[62]

Unlike the other non-naturals, however, there are some difficulties in applying it to animals. The reason for this is simply that there was an on-going debate during the early modern period as to whether animals actually experienced emotions. The seventh century scholar Isidore of Seville stated that horses were 'the only creature that weeps for man and feels the emotion of grief'. In the twelfth century Albertus Magnus argued that they share traits such as 'knowledge, habits (that is, good or bad customary behaviour), fear, boldness ... concupiscence, desire,

---

[59] F. Sofford, A new almanack (London, 1621), sig. B7v ; J. Woodhouse, A new almanacke and prognostication (London, 1634), sig. B6r.and R. French, 'Astrology in medical practice' in L. Garcia-Ballester, R. French, J. Arrizabalaga and A. Cunnigham (eds) Practical Medicine from Salerno to the Black Death (Cambridge, 1999), pp. 30–59.

[60] W. Vaughn, Directions for Health both Naturall and Artificiall (London, 1617), pp. 229–230.

[61] R. Porter, Flesh in the Age of Reason (London, 2003), p. 47.

[62] N. Culpeper, Galen's Art, p. 132 and C. Rawcliffe, Medicine & Society, p. 10.

wrath and the like with humans.[63] Other medieval authors held that animals lacked the ability to 'reason' which meant that they were unable to make rational decisions. It therefore followed that animals were only able to behave instinctively.[64] That said, by the seventeenth century there were many people who believed that animals did have passions and emotions. Gervase Markham argued that horses 'have sense and feeling of Affections as namely, to Love, to Hate, to be Angry, to Rejoyce, to be Sorry, and to Fear'. As Keith Thomas had pointed out, such sentiments were part of an increasing tendency to credit animals with 'reason, intelligence, language and almost every other human quality'.[65]

Whether one agrees that animals could feel emotions, there is one form of 'passion' that could sometimes be manipulated. Both male and female animals were thought to have strong sexual urges. Bulls were said to 'burn in Lust' and cows were also said to be very lustful, 'and doe most eagerly desire the company of their male'. However, according to Gervase Markham, goats had the most 'lusty constitution' which 'exceeds all other cattel'. That said, Markham warned readers that the sexual activities of all working animals needed to be restricted 'for nothing sooner shortens life in any Creature'.[66] Castration, which was the most dramatic and permanent way of controlling this activity was also believed to produce healthier animals. Another benefit for the owner was that it also made the beast easier to control.[67]

Conclusion

Preventative health care was one of the basic tenets of popular medicine in early modern England. The concept that it was better to retain health rather than fight illness was one based on tradition, observation and good sense. While much literature initially seems to focus exclusively on human health, Information on how to provide one's animals with a health lifestyle was widely available both through the oral and

---

[63] E. Brehaut, *An Encyclopedist of the Dark Ages: Isidore of Seville* (New York, 1912), p. 144; M. Albertus, *On Animals: A Medieval Zoological Summary*, Vol I, (trans) Kitchell, K.F. and I.M Resnick (Baltimore, 1999), p. 606.

[64] J.E. Salisbury, *The Beast Within: Animals in the Middle Ages* (London, 1994), p. 5.

[65] G. Markham, *Maister-piece*, p. 15 and K. Thomas, *Man and the Natural World*, pp. 128–9.

[66] G. Markham, *A way to get wealth* (London, 1648), p. 122; E. Toppsell, *Foure-Footed Beastes*, sig. G1v and 172 and G. Markham, *Complete jockey*, p. 41.

[67] K. Thomas, *Man and the Natural World*, p. 93.

the print cultures. This focused on the Galenic non-naturals, which were things 'necessary for the Preservation of Health, but hurt it when ill applied'.[68]

A recent work by Sandra Dolby suggests that the popularity of modern 'self-help' books lies with the fact that they offer readers 'a focused meditation on how they might best act with prudence in their individual lives'. Dolby suggests that although authors generally claim that their information is 'new', it actually almost always contains 'whatever [advice] is useful from the past'.[69] In fact, modern ideas of good health regimens are extremely similar to those of medieval and early modern England. While the underlying theory of why illness occurs has changed, the practical advice has been, and still is, based on the foundation of clean air, good diet, sufficient sleep, exercise and the maintenance of stable emotions. Presumably, the way in which early modern writers used these categories to offer information in manageable, easily understood segments meant that they also sounded like wise guidelines to contemporary readers.

It seems highly unlikely people believed that attempts to maintain a state of good health both for themselves and their animals could always keep illness at bay. However, I think that the emphasis on trying to protect the health of one's animals served two purposes. In the first place, adherence to all or even only some of the non-naturals probably did result in stronger bodies that were more resistant to disease. In fact, many of them are still recognised as building blocks of good health in the twenty-first century. Secondly, I would argue that being provided with, and attempting to follow, a systematic method of preventative health served an important function. It addressed what has been recognised as the rampant feeling of helplessness in the face of disease.[70] Domesticated animals were even more helpless, being totally dependent on the humans who cared for them. There were both economic and moral reasons for humans to want to protect the health of their animals. Perhaps, trying to provide their charges with a good lifestyle provided people with the feeling of even a small sense of control over their health, the animals future and that of their own family.

---

[68] J. Pechey, *A Plain Introduction to the Art of Physick* (London, 1697), p. 59.

[69] S. K. Dolby, *Self-Help Books: Why Americans Keep Reading Them* (Champaign, 2005), pp. xi and 14.

[70] K. Thomas, *Religion and the Decline of Magic* (London, 1991), p. 17.

CHAPTER SIX

REMEDIAL MEDICINE

> Now notwithstanding all a mans carefulnesse, beasts daylie doe get
> infirmities, and often fall into mortall extremities.[1]

As Gervase Markham, and many other authors, reminded their readers, no matter how carefully owners tried to protect the health of their
animals, such efforts would not always work. Although there were
many reasons as to why this was the case, most were due at least in part
to the effects of domestication. Unlike those living in the wild, the
health of working animals lay almost entirely in the hands of their owners or care-takers. Those who chose to overwork or 'over-hunt' their
charges, particularly in poor weather conditions, were likely to cause a
'weakness or poorness of body' which would result in 'some disease or
the other'. Failing to provide clean, dry housing in which they could
rest after their labour or providing insufficient or poor quality food
could also lead to illness.[2]

Animals could also succumb to disease because of the sinful behaviour of humans. Although it was believed that they were incapable of
guilt or committing sin, animals were seen as a conduit through which
humans who displeased God by their behaviour or thoughts could be
punished.[3] This could be manifested through God's 'three mortall
arrows' of pestilence, famine or war. Pestilence might appear in the
form of a 'cattle plague' or while all species might suffer starvation
because of extreme, unseasonable crop failures. Another way for the
deity to punish humans was to cause either chronic or acute illnesses
on their animals.

This chapter will examine the various types of therapeutic treatments
and medicines that were recommended for sick animals in early modern
England. Although 'therapeutics' comes from the Greek 'iattend', which

---

[1] G. Markham, *Cheape and Good Husbandry* (London, 1614), p. 46.
[2] C. Estienne, *Maison rustique, or The countrey farme* (London, 1616), p. 677 and
A.S. *The husbandman, farmer and grasier's compleat instructor* (1697), p. 15.
[3] W. Dade, *The Country-mans Kalendar* (London, 1684), sig. B3r; T. Tryon, *The
countryman's companion* (London, 1688), sig. A2v and A. Walsham, *Providence in Early
Modern England* (Oxford, 2001), pp. 156–7.

means to heal or treat, in this period the term was used to cover all matters related to the science or art of healing.[4] This included the non-naturals discussed in the previous chapter, as well as materia medica and physical or surgical treatments. The aim of all of these was to redress the imbalance of humours that was making the animal ill. There were two main ways of doing this, depending on whether an excess or a deficiency of a humour needed to be addressed. Both methods could involve a range of organic and/or inorganic ingredients that could be used either internally or externally, as well a range of 'physical' or mechanical methods to remove excess humours or impurities from the body.

The ways in which diseases would be diagnosed and treated are documented in a vast range of early modern texts. Andrew Wear has suggested that, for the most part, the therapies mirrored those used by the author and their own families.[5] This is certainly true to some degree, mainly within the underlying theories of how health and illness affected all living creatures. However, there were a number of differences related to who the patient was. These could be found both in the way in which disease was diagnosed, in the types of recommended treatments and their quantities and ingredients. The first was obviously based on the fact that, unlike humans, animals were unable to verbalise their symptoms which meant that a diagnosis would be based most heavily on visible signs. While there were thought to be many similarities between human and animal anatomy, the numerous types of domesticated beasts came in a range of sizes and shapes. This meant that treatments might need to be altered for specific animals, although one argued that since 'the body of the great cattel is, so is the body of the lesser cattel, almost of like nature ... there is a small difference betwixt their medicines & betwixt their diseases'.[6] That said, certain considerations such as whether an animal was an herbivore or carnivore, as well as whether it was meant for worker or a 'comforter' (ie lap dog) appear to have resulted in variations in the actual ingredients and the quantities that needed to be use for different types of creatures.

Before discussing the types of remedial treatments used for animals, the following section will begin by examining the ways in which

---

[4] W.J. Dilling, *Bruce and Dilling's Materia Medica and Therapeutics* (London, 1933), p. 2.

[5] A. Wear, 'Making Sense of Health and the Environment in Early Modern England' in A. Wear (ed.) *Medicine in Society: Historical Essays* (Cambridge, 1992), p. 144.

[6] A. Snape, *The anatomy of a horse* (London, 1683), sig. A3r and L. Mascal, *The Government of Cattle* (London, 1662) p. 213.

diseases were diagnosed as either 'inward' or 'outward'.[7] It will then move on to the two main ways of dealing with a humoural imbalance. The first was by replenishing a deficit by introducing substances meant to be retained in order to 'comforte ... the chiefe officiall Members of the Body'. These would differ depending on the humour in question and whether the patient needed to be cooled, heated, moistened or dried.[8] Removing or 'taking away' excess humours or substances involved purges which worked either through urine, faeces, mucus, sweat, pus or blood. In some cases this would involve ingesting remedies that had diuretic or laxative properties. It was also possible to apply irritants to the skin to cause blistering, as well as using surgical instruments to let blood. The final section will consider 'chyrugical' or surgical treatments, which carried a number of risks and were best only attempted when other methods had failed.

Diagnosis

The first step in any remedial process was to determine the nature of the illness and to decide whether it was an 'inward' or 'outward' malady. For human patients, a modern consultation generally includes listening to a narrative of the course of their illness. Martin Kemp has argued that diagnosis has always been 'intimately linked' to visible signs or 'how someone looks'.[9] This is undoubtedly true in many cases, particularly when broken bones, skin ulcers or other 'physical' signs can be seen. However, in the largest number of cases actual disease labels are only produced after the study of samples of bodily fluids such as blood or urine.

Modern diagnosis for animals also includes both visible signs and clinical tests. In the early modern period, the process was typically a mixture of observation and examination of various forms of excreta. Of course, in a society where animals and humans lived and worked so closely together, it seems likely that even slight changes in the physical appearance of an animal would be readily noticed. For example, a

---

[7] Anon, *The Perfect Husbandman, or The Art of Husbandry* (London, 1657), p. 227.

[8] D. LeClerc, *The History of Physick, or an Account of the Rise and Progress of the Art* (London, 1699), p. 195 and T. Cocke, *Kitchin-Physick: or, Advice to the Poor, By Way of Dialogue* (London, 1676), p. 9.

[9] M. Kemp, 'Medicine in View: Art and Visual Representation' in I. Loudon (ed) *Western Medicine: An Illustrated History* (Oxford, 1997), pp. 12/1–22.

healthy ram or ewe was expected to have eyes which looked 'large, black and glistening with golden colour'. Rather than having a nose damp as 'Dew-water', a sick creature would 'be dry on the top of his nose'.[10]

Lay healers could also use the charts included in a number of texts to help put a name to the affliction. Figure 6.1 dates from 1616 and shows an oxen surrounded are illnesses or injuries that affected particular parts of the body. On the left side is a list of general disorders, or ones that affected internal organs. In order to aid the reader, page numbers where further information can be found were also included.

Figure 6.2 is an even more elaborate and detailed illustration of a horse. Printed in 1679, this is a very decorative image spread over two pages. This would have been an extremely expensive image to either produce or purchase second-hand, and would have driven up the price of the book accordingly.[11] It is fortunate that the Wellcome Library's copy has survived intact, as many contemporary texts are missing comparable illustrations. For example, their edition of James Lambert, *The countrymans* [sic] *treasure*, 1683 is missing the frontispiece which is a particularly attractive portrait of a cow, a bull and a pig.[12] The most likely explanation is that the images were removed from books in order to hang them on walls for both decorative and/or practical purposes.

Another way of diagnosing animals was through the study of their excreta. Blood, urine or dung were all thought to contain the 'superfluities' or 'bad humours' which caused disease. A sample of blood, for example, could be examined before, during and after it coagulated. This could be done using different senses, including sight, taste and texture. Contemporary texts on animal health suggest that the examination of urine or dung was more common than that of blood. As with blood, samples could be analysed by its colour, quality and smell.[13]

One of the most detailed descriptions of uroscopy can be found in Gervase Markham's works, which first appeared in the early seventeenth century and continued to be reissued in various editions through the 1730's. A healthy horse was expected to have 'pale, whitish, yellow .... somewhat strong smelling urine'. If it were 'extraordinary

[10] M. Harward, *The Herds-man's Mate, Or, a Guide for Herds-men* (Dublin, 1673), p. 12.

[11] T. Watt, *Cheap Print and Popular Piety, 1550–1640* (Cambridge, 1996), p. 262.

[12] Wellcome Library 34024/A and J. Lambert, *The countrymans treasure* (London, 1683).

[13] N.G. Siraisi, *Medieval & Early Renaissance Medicine* (Chicago, 1990), pp. 124–5 and C. Rawcliffe, *Medicine and Society in Later Medieval England* (Stroud, 1995), pp. 47–8.

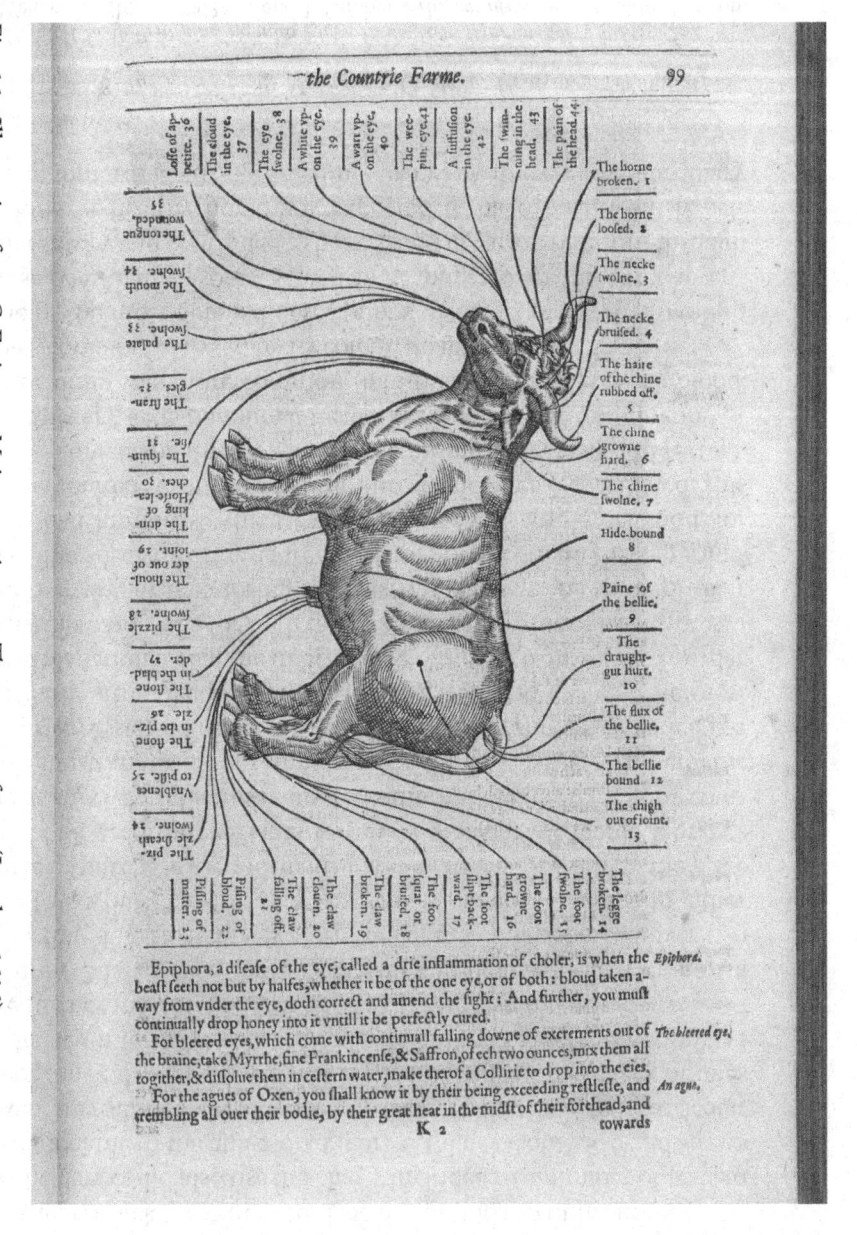

Fig. 6.1. Illustration from C. Estienne, *Maison rustique*, or *The country farme* (London, 1616). Courtesy of the Wellcome Library, London.

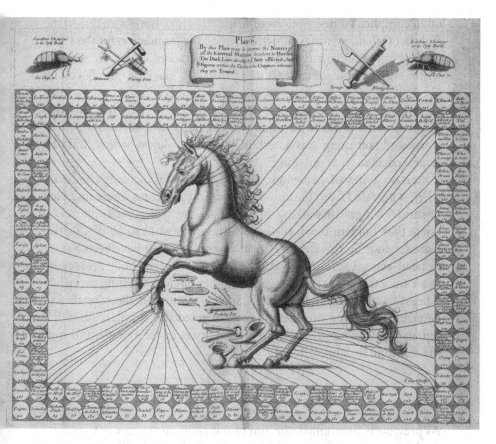

Fig. 6.2. Illustration from J. de Solleysel, *The compleat horseman* (London, 1679). Courtesy of the Wellcome Library, London.

White … creamy' it signified that the beast might be 'subject to the Stone and the stopping of the Kidneys'. Pale green urine, on the other hand, was linked to a 'Weak Back, and consumption of the Seed', while black urine signified that the 'Horse sickness is Mortal and hardly to be preserved by any Physick'.[14]

Other excretions, such as dung, were also useful for diagnostic purposes. Although Gervase Markham was a proponent of uroscopy, he argued that dung was 'no less worthy of Note than the Urine'.[15] That said, the guidelines on dung appear very simplistic compared to the

---

[14] G. Markham, *Markham's Maister-piece* (London, 1683), p. 25 and Anon, *The experienced jockey* (1684), p. 80.
[15] Ibid.

often complicated descriptions of urine. This may have been due to the fact that Galenic writings, which provided the foundation for the study of the bodily fluids, included urine but not faeces. One early modern writer, for example, stated that dung that was 'black or muddy colour, like Pellets, yet hot and greasy' signaled 'foul feeding'. Hard, reddish excrements suggested that the horse had been 'over-heated' or 'over-strained'. Since a healthy animal was expected to void 'round pellets', 'loose and soft dung' was a certain sign of 'weakness' which must 'be remedied as soon as possible.[16]

Certain types of behaviour also suggested problems, particularly when it deviated from the animals' usual way of acting. These included posture, changes in walking or feeding. One typical example was a horse that 'holdeth down his head, which was wont to be of cheerful Countenance'. In this case, a typical diagnosis would have been a fever or head-ache. A fever could also be diagnosed by the body and breath of an animal being excessively hot. Another obvious warning was when a beast would 'forsake his meat'.[17] Such signs helped the caretaker to determine the type of illness, how it affected the animal's humoural imbalance, whether it needed remedial drugs or treatments, and how these should be administered.

Remedial Medicine: 'a putting to'

As previously mentioned, the aim of remedial medicine was to redress the humoural imbalance which was causing the illness. There were two main therapeutic methods for attempting to do this. The first involved introducing substances meant to be retained in the body in order to boost the deficiency of a particular humour, or humours. This process was generally begun by determining an appropriate diet supplemented by appropriate medicinal potions.[18] Of course, there was a fine line between food and 'drugs', as many of the latter contained ingredients which might also fall into the first category. This became especially true

---

[16] N. Cox, *The gentleman's recreation: in four parts* (London, 1697), p. 80 and G.L. *The Gentleman's new jockey: or, Farrier's approved guide* (London, 1691), pp. 39–40.

[17] J.H. *The gentleman's jockey and approved farrier* (London,1683) p. 41; G. Markham, *Master-piece revived*, p. 18; J. Lambert, *The country-man's treasure: shewing the nature, causes, and cure of all diseases incident to cattle, viz. oxen, cows, calves* (London, 1703), p. 49 and R. Gardner, *Veterinarium Meteorologist Astrology* (London, 1698), sig. A2v.

[18] T. Cocke, *Kitchen-Physick: or, Advice to the Poor, By Way of Dialogue* (1676), p. 9.

when treating domesticated animals, the majority of whom were vegetarians.

Plants, in common with animals, had innate qualities of heat, coldness, wetness and dryness. According to Galenic theory this meant that cool, wet foods could be used to treat hot, dry diseases or the opposite for cold, wet illnesses. Some of these were also thought to thicken the humours, while others thinned them in order to help the body excrete them. The first consideration was to determine the nature of which of these properties pertained to an item. This was followed by deciding on the quantities to be used in what were delineated in 'medicinall diets'. These included 'thinning' or 'sparing' or 'liberall or full' diets, as well as 'a meane diet betwixt both'. There were a range of considerations that had to be taken in account when determining which would be most suitable. The first was the nature of the illness and of the patient, followed by the time of the year, the weather and the region where the patient lived.[19] In theory, such diets could be used for all living creatures. However, the most frequent references to 'medicinall diets' in popular medical literature apply to humans, rather than domesticated animals. Despite this, there were still a great deal of advice in texts that provided basic guidelines for feeding different types of sick animals as 'proper food and nursing will much facilitate the cure'. In many cases, it is also possible to decipher the basic format of a 'spare', 'full' or 'in-between diet' for different types of cattle. If the illness was linked to an excess of food, the recommended therapy was to severely restrict these supplies as part of a 'spare' diet. Such advice was probably based on the observation that many poorly animals, when left to their own devices, would reduce their intake or even attempt to 'cure themselves by abstinence'.[20] Although most authors did not recommend starving sick animals, one argued that fasting was desirable as the quickest means of purging 'the Load of crude and undigested Aliment which is in the paunch'.[21]

---

[19] J.V. Nutton, *Ancient Medicine* (London, 2004), p. 241; H.J. Cook, 'Good Advice and Little Medicine: The Professional Advice of Early Modern English Physicians', *Journal of British Studies*, 33 (1994), pp. 14–17; M. Grant, *Galen on Food and Diet* (London, 2000), p. 11; K. Albala, *Food in Early Modern Europe* (Westport, Conn., 2003), p. 216 and M. O'Hara-May, 'Food or Medicines?', *Transactions of the British Society for the History of Pharmacy*, 1 (1971), p. 65.

[20] E. Gayton, *The art of longevity, or, a diaeticall institution* (1659), p. 5.

[21] J. Barker, *An account of the present epidemical distemper amongst the black cattle* (London, 1745), p. 16.

A 'full' diet, on the other hand, was best used when an animal was 'weake or sicke'. There appear to have been two main factors in determining what this should consist of based on the type of animal and its perceived worth. Most domesticated animals were vegetarian, with the exception of dogs. This meant, in general, that most would simply have received greater quantities of their normal food. Although dogs are carnivorous, the daily diet for many would have been 'bread made of a third part of wheate, a third part of barley, and a third part of rye, because that being so mixt it keepeth them faire and fat'. Despite these perceived benefits, a warm, cooked mixture of boiled sheep entrails, or other offal, might be mixed with their meal in order to make it even more nutritious.[22]

Since the majority of domesticated animals were not carnivores, however, other equally wholesome ingredients needed to be substituted. In many examples this took the form of wine or beer. Galen was attributed with saying that wine 'nourisheth above all other aliment', a concept expounded by many early modern writers. The most nourishing wines were red ones which were generally thick and sweet. Yellow or 'white' wines could be substituted, but were thought to be less effective for building up a body weakened by disease.[23] While a human diet might include imbibing sweet wines on their own, those for animals tended to include it as a base, or core ingredient in remedies. In addition to being a specific colour, each type had a range of other characteristics which included sweetness, 'heat', 'thickness' or 'thin-ness'. As a result, this meant that certain types were best suited to specific kinds of illnesses. The humoural constitution of red wine was generally thought to be 'cold', although some were 'moist' while others were 'dry'. Rich wines which were thick and sweet, such as sack, were particularly effective at building up bodies weakened by disease. 'Small' or weaker white wines were hotter substances and useful for were good for 'loosening the belly' Yellow wines, on the other hand, were considered to be 'the hottest' wines and were therefore of greatest use to treat cold, wet diseases.[24]

---

[22] C. Estienne, *Maison rustique*, p 677 and H. Peachem, *The Complete Gentleman, The Truth of our Times, and The Art of Living in London* (London, 1622), p. 238.

[23] T. Whitaker, *The Tree of Humane Life, or, The Bloud of the Grape* (London, 1638), p. 24 and W. Vaughn, *Directions for Health, both Naturall and Artificiall* (London, 1617), p. 43.

[24] J. Hart, *Klinike, or The Diet of the Diseased* (London, 1633), p. 120 and W. Turner, *A new boke of the natures and properties of all wines that are commonly used here in England* (London, c.1568), sig. D7v.

In a broad sense, 'cattle' such as oxen were thought to have a cooler constitution than horses. This supports the suitability of a remedy consisting of walnuts and hard cheese, 'tempered' in thick (red) wine. This is an interesting combination, as in moderation, cheese was thought to 'engender good bloud'. Nuts were hot and dry in the second degree if 'drye', although cold and moist when new. Lovell fails to specify what type of nut should be used, perhaps leaving it up to his readers to decide on whether the beast was suffering from a 'cold' or 'hot' illness. A similar recipe for weak cattle was based on 'gall nuts', apples and wheat beaten together and steeped in three pints of red wine. In this case, the wine would have helped to build up the body while the cold and watery nature of the apples would help to re-hydrate it.[25]

Horses, on the other hand, required 'colder' remedies. According to the humoural theory, this meant that they were theoretically most likely to suffer from hot diseases, such as fevers. As a result, 'cold' ingredients such as 'yellow' wine were considered to be particularly suitable for horses. One author suggested a cordial for weak horses based on thin white wine mixed with 'two ounces of Hony' to make it more palatable. Another earlier text suggested a more savoury mixture for poorly horses, consisting of a 'pottage made of a pint of Wine, stamped Garlicke, and tenne whites of egges'.[26]

Due to the relatively high cost of wine through most of the early modern period, it seems likely that sour or otherwise spoiled wines would have been using in animal remedies. As one translator of a French text noted, 'our Author ...liv'd in a Wine Country, commonly prescribes Wine for a Vehicle: But in this Country that affords Ale, we may make use of it instead of Wine'.[27] Both beer and ale, being much cheaper, were frequently called for in popular veterinary texts. Both drinks consisted of malted barley, although they could be concocted from wheat, rye or even oatmeal. The major difference between the two was that, after the 1520's, hops were added during the manufacturing process of beer. There were many different types of each drink, with the cheapest and least alcoholic being referred to as 'small beer'. This drink

[25] W. Lovell, *The Dukes desk newly broken up: Wherein is discovered Divers Rare Recipts of Physick and Surgery* (London, 1661), p. 95; M. Harward, *The Herds-man's Mate*, p. 25; Swallow, *An Almanack* (Cambridge, 1662), sig. C2r and Dove, *An Almanack* (Cambridge, 1638), sig C6r.

[26] J. Halfpenny, *The gentlemans jockey and approved farrier* (London, 1676), p. 194 and C. Estienne, *Maison rustique*, p. 137.

[27] J. de Solleysel, *The compleat horseman* (London, 1692), sig. 3v.

was found in most households, being widely consumed by both adults and children. At the other end of the category was the much more powerful and expensive 'strong beer' which was seen as a more 'democratic alternative' to small beer for those who could not afford wine.[28]

In medical usage, beer was often recommended as being better than ale, due to the hops which were able to 'cleanseth the bloud from all corrupt humours'.[29] It also provided an excellent base to which other ingredients could be added to, or steeped in. On the other hand, ale was widely recognised as being highly nutritious and useful for building up sick animals. Gervase Markham recommended soaking oats, which would have been the normal fare for horses, in ale.[30] A more complicated recipe involved boiling nutmeg and tar in strong ale. This was then meant to be fed to poorly horses 'two spoonfuls at a time, using it several times with two days distance between each time'.[31]

Once the core liquid was chosen, there were a wide variety of herbs and other organic materials that could be added. Unlike the modern tendency to delineate 'food' from 'medicine', during the early modern period the two terms were often used interchangeably. Aniseeds, for example, were an extremely popular flavouring in bread or biscuits and were also coated in sugar candy to take as a breath freshener. Furthermore, the seeds were hot and dry, which meant that they were a useful ingredient in a potion to dry up sores in horses' noses.[32]

The use of only one main ingredient was known as a 'simple', while more complex remedies were referred to as 'compound' mixtures.[33] In technical terms, each medicine was thought to have two dominant qualities, the 'active' and the 'passive'. The former was broken down into either hot or cold and the former into dry or wet, with the strength being further quantified on a scale from temperate (neutral) to the fourth degree. Mathematical skills would certainly have been needed

---

[28] J.M. Bennett, *Ale, Beer, and Brewsters in England: Women's Work in a Changing World 1300–1600* (Oxford, 1996), pp. 8–9 and L. Hill Curth and T. Cassidy, 'Medical Constructions of Wine and Beer in Early Modern England' in A. Smyth (ed) *A Pleasing Sinne: Drink Conviviality in Seventeenth Century England* (Woodbridge, 2004), pp. 143–159.

[29] T. Venner, *Via recta ad vitam longam* (London, 1638), p. 44.

[30] G. Markham, *A Discourse of horsmanshippe* (London, 1593), p. 45.

[31] *The Shepherd's Almanac*, (London, 1675) sig. C6r and 1678, sig. C6r.

[32] K. Albala, *Food in Early Modern Europe* (Westport, Connecticut, 2003), p. 42 and H. Best, *The Farming and memorandum Books of Henry Best of Elmswell*, 1642 (Oxford, 1984), p. 200.

[33] M.J. Dobson, *Contours of Death and Disease in Early Modern England* (Cambridge, 1997), p. 265.

to calculate the correct dosage of a compound drug, given the increasing number of variables. John Henry has illustrated this problem with the example of a medicine containing sandalwood and honey. Since sandalwood was considered cold and wet in the second degree, a dram could only be 'neutralised' by two ounces, rather than a single dram of honey which was hot and dry in the second degree.[34]

The majority of people who cared for sick animals, however, were not mathematicians interested in the finer intricacies of calculating dosages and most writers provided straightforward, easy to understand and follow recipes. Based on Galenic principles, most remedies assumed a strong relationship between the symbolic properties of herbs, and their empirical effects. One of the main principles, called the 'Doctrine of Signatures', was based on the idea that all plants offered either visual or other clues as to their medicinal qualities. It therefore followed, for example, that yellow flowers could be used to treat jaundice. Similarly, herbs that grew on stones, such as parsley-piert were thought to dissolve kidney stones. This also carried over to similarities between different types of animal matter. Therefore, in theory, the lung of a fox could be used to treat lung disease in man.[35] Although 'stale urine' or dried faeces from a human was sometimes called for as a base for other ingredients, I have been unable to find any examples, however, of parts of humans being used to treat animals.

Closely linked to the Doctrine of Signatures were the principles of 'sympathy' and 'antipathy'. The first rested on the idea that diseases caused by a specific planet could be cured by herbs 'astrally' linked to it, which were gathered 'at the right Planetary hours'. At the most basic level, this meant that 'herbs and plant under the dominion of the Sun' should be gathered on Sunday, those linked to the Moon on Monday, Mars on Tuesday and so on.[36] The principles of antipathy recommended using vegetable matter linked to the planet opposite to the one causing the disease.

---

[34] A. Bragman, 'Alligation Alternate and the Composition of Medicines: Arithmetic and Medicine in Early Modern England', Medical History, 49 (2005), pp. 293–320 and J. Henry, 'Doctors and healers', pp. 191–221.

[35] R. Porter, The Greatest Benefit to Mankind: A Medical History of Humanity from Antiquity to the Present (London, 1997), p. 134; Raphael, Raphael's Medical Astrology: The Effects of the Planets and Signs upon the Human Body (London, 1937), p. 68; R. Mabey, Flora Britannica Book of Wild Herbs (London, 1998), p. 105 and D. Guthrie, A History of Medicine (London, 1960), p. 160.

[36] J. Blagrave, Blagrave's Astrological Practice of Physick (London, 1689), sig. A6r and p. 12.

Keith Thomas has commented that 'scientific opinion' was increasingly negative towards the idea of 'sympathy' during the later seventeenth century.[37] According to Mary Lindemann, 'sympathetic cures' along with other astrologically related treatments continued to be widely used well into the eighteenth century.[38] Such statements illustrate the vast difference between 'popular' medical texts, and lay beliefs and what was happening in the sphere of the 'educated elite'. As discussed in Chapter 4, the majority of popular medical texts continued to provide time honoured, conservative medical advice through the early modern period. Very few writers even touched upon the model developed by Paracelsus, whom John Henry has referred to as one of the 'earliest subscribers of ontological medicine'. Paracelsian medicine rested on the belief that God had endowed all animate and non-animate things, including diseases, with their own divine spark or 'archeus'. In order to treat someone who had been 'attacked' by disease, it was necessary to determine which drug had an archeus paralleling that of the patient's illness. Unlike traditional Galenic remedies, Paracelsian remedies relied on the elements of salt, sulphur and mercury. Both Henry and Andrew Wear have suggested that it was these chemical ingredients, rather than Paraclesian theory itself, that were popularized, a theory which is supported by a range of primary source material.[39]

Many recipes for animals, for example, included remedies based on a combination of Galenic and Paracelsian ingredients. As a hot, drying ingredient, 'treacle' combined with either herbs or spices were thought to energise or revive poorly animals. One author suggested that, in addition to a 'wholesome strong' diet, 'foundrig' (ie foundering) horses should be given a drink made up of 'a quart of Ale boiled with Pepper and Cinnamon and an ounce of London treacle'. Sick cattle could be given a mixture of plaintain and treacle mixed in a quart of ale and sheep could be given 'one pennyworth of Treacle' mixed with a bit of

---

[37] E.G. Wheelwright, *The Physick Garden* (London, 1934), p. 147 and K. Thomas, *Man and the Natural World: Changing Attitudes in England 1500–1800* (London, 1983), p. 84.

[38] M. Lindemann, *Medicine and Society in Early Modern Europe* (Cambridge, 1999), p. 21.

[39] J. Henry, 'Doctors and healers: popular culture and the medical profession' in (ed) S. Pumfrey, P.L. Rossi and M. Slawinski (eds) *Science, culture and popular belief in Renaissance Europe* (Manchester, 1991), pp. 191–221 ; A.G. Debus, 'Chemists, Physicians and Changing Perspectives on the Scientific Revolution', *ISIS*, 89, No. 1 (March 1998), 66–91 and A. Wear, *Knowledge & Practice in English Medicine 1550–1680*, (Cambridge, 2000), p. 39.

'tumerick' and 'English Saffron'. Alternatively, a drink of treacle, hemp-seed, ivy and elder leaves along with 'fetherfew' [feverfew] could be offered.[40] One recipe for a purging mixture suggested boiling worm-wood and celedine in strong beer, before adding honey, butter and Venice treacle.[41]

'Treacle' was an opium based medicine, which had been widely used since the middle ages to treat sleeping problems, pain and to improve moods. The *Pharmacopopoeia Londinensis*, first published in 1618, included a number of medicines based on opium, such as theriac, which came from the Latin word for antidote and was later corrupted to 'trea-cle', mithridite, mecoium and diacodium. This was considered to be an extremely strong medicine, 'perhaps the most powerful [medicine] that has been hitherto known'.[42] There were many different recipes for pre-paring treacle, most of which contained between thirty and fifty ingre-dients, in addition to molasses. Most people were likely to purchase treacle ready-made, however, in order to avoid having to find rather unusual ingredients such as 'the horn of a stag' or 'flesh of vipers'.[43]

The quantities administered seem to be at least loosely based on the size of the animal in question. Potions for greater cattle were usually measured in quarts, while those for dogs might be based on pints.[44] However, the main differences between the types of medicines used depended on the type of illness and the ultimate aim of the therapy. At the lowest level, it needed to be determined whether an animal had an 'internal' or 'external' illness. The former were those that were 'bred within the body', as opposed to those which 'communicate with the outward parts'.[45] It was then necessary to determine whether the cure

---

[40] S. Strangehopes, *The book of knowledge* (London, 1701), pp. 115–6; J. Lambert, *The country-man's treasure* (London, 1703), pp. 36–7 and R. Gardner, *Veterinarium Meteorologist Astrology* (London, 1698), sig. A3r.

[41] W. Dade, *The Countryman's Calendar* (Cambridge, 1698) sig. B3v.

[42] W. O. Schalick III, 'To Market, to Market: The Theory and Practice of Opiates in the Middle Ages' in M.L. Meldrum (ed) *Opiods and Pain Relief: A Historical Perspective* (Seattle, 2003), pp. 5–20; A. Sala, *Opiologia: or, A treatise concerning the nature...of opium*, (trans) T. Bretnor (London, 1618), sig. A4v; B. Hodgson, *In the Arms of Morpheus: The Tragic History of Laudanum, Morphine, and Patent Medicines* (Buffalo, N.Y. 2001), pp. 18, 24 and J. Pechey, *A collection of chronical diseases* (London, 1692), p. 63.

[43] W. Brockbank, 'Sovereign Remedies: A Critical Depreciation of the seventeenth century London Pharmacoepia', *Medical History*, 8 (1964), 1–14 and B. Hodgson, *In the Arms of Morpheus: the Tragic History of Laudanum, Morphine and Patent Medicines* (Buffalo, N.Y., 2001), p. 19.

[44] G. Markham, *Markham's Methode or Epitome* (London, 1633) p. 60.

[45] Ibid., *Markham's Master-piece revived* (London, 1681), p. 29.

could be affected by purging the system in order to 'take away' excess humours or through retaining the remedial potion within the body. 'External' or visible diseases or injuries will be discussed in the final part of this chapter.

Remedial Medicine: 'a taking away'

The second main form of remedial medicine was based on 'disburdening' the body of 'corrupt and superfluous' matter in order to bring the humours back into equilibrium.[46] In general, these worked by purging the bodies through various orifices. These included diuretic potions or suppositories to provoke urine or faeces. There were also a range of medicines to cause vomiting, sneezing, coughing or sweating. Physical procedures were also widely used, such as bloodletting or baths to 'wash' excess humours from the body.

For humans, the type of purging method chosen would depend on a range of factors which included the time of the year, the temperature, what part of the body was affected and by which humour, the strength of the patient and the potential treatment and the place and configuration of the moon.[47] It does not appear from available evidence, however, that all of these considerations were taken into account for sick animals. Popular texts suggest that it was more common to begin by considering the nature of the imbalance, and what part of the body needed to be treated. Linked to this was the need to determine whether to use 'external' or 'internal' purgations. Sometimes ailments, such as a horse being full of 'grease and foul matter' required more than one type of purge. John Halfpenny recommended that such horses be treated first with 'sharp exercise to dissolve and melt the foulness' followed by 'strong scowrings to bring it away in abundance'.[48] The second part of his treatment involved what were also referred to as 'frictions'. This will involve preparing a hot mixture of ingredients which would be rubbed into the sick animal. One recipe for sick horses involved heating up a batch of vinegar and patch-grease which was massaged into the animals' body 'against the hair'.[49]

---

[46] R. Allestree, *An almanacke* (London,1640), sig. C5r.
[47] T. Bretnor, *A new almanacke* (London, 1609), sig. B3r.
[48] J. Halfpenny, *The gentlemans jockey, and approved farrier* (London, 1676), p. 53.
[49] G. Markham, *Cheape and good*, (1614), p. 73.

Since the humors were thought to 'move from the inward parts of the body to the outward' as the moon moved from full to a quarter, it was better to use the external purgations during the first and third weeks of the moons course and save internal ones for the other weeks.[50] Drugs taken either to purge or 'comfort' the body would also react in different ways according to the movements of the stars and planets. If administered in the 'wrong hour', they would have the opposite effect from what they were meant to do. This was particularly true of medicines given under signs that 'chew the cud', such Aries and Taurus, as the patient would be unable to keep from vomiting them up. If the aim was to purge the body, then the most auspicious time to take a purgation would be when the Moon was in an aspect with a moist planet, such as Cancer, Scorpio or Pisces, which 'stirred up and down' the humours, which would aid in the process.[51]

According to one author, medicinal purges for animals consisted either of pills or potions. The former were described as 'any solid and substantiall stuffe fixed together ... being made into round balles' which 'are cast downe the horses'. It was thought that the best time to administer pills was in the watery sign of Pisces, which would help to dissolve completely in the body. Potions, on the other hand, consisted of 'any liquid purging matter to drinke, whether it be purging powders dissolued in Wine or Ale ... [or]any other liquid stuffe. The former were to 'cleane the head and braine' while the latter were meant to cleanse the stomacke, guts, and euery other inward member'. It was believed that the most auspicious time to take such a purgation was when the Moon was in an aspect with a moist planet, such as Cancer, Scorpio or Pisces, which 'stirred up and down' the humours, which would aid in the process. If given in the 'wrong [astrological] hour, they might give the opposite effect from what they were meant to do. This was particularly true of medicines given under signs that 'chew the cud', such Aries and Taurus, as the animal would be unable to keep from vomiting them up.[52]

There were a wide range of purging medicines for animals, most of which were based on herbal or other organic ingredients. Some authors

---

[50] G. Gilden, *A new almanacke* (London, 1616), sig. C3r.
[51] J. Blagrave, *Blagrave's Astrological Practice of Physick* (London, 1687), sig. A5r and R. Clark, *Clark an almanack* (London, 1634), sig. C2r.
[52] J. Blagrave, *Blagrave's Astrological* sig. A5r; Swallow, *An Almanack* (Cambridge, 1640), sig. B8r and G. Markham, *Markham's Maister-piece* (London, 1615), p. 197.

recommended periodically taking dogs to 'any place where the grass or green corn grows luxuriant', so that they could have the opportunity to rid themselves of 'any thing offensive upon their stomachs'. A simple suggestions for 'cleansing and purging' horses involved feeding them 'Sodden Barley' or putting 'a little Rye in the sheaf'.[53] Another 'general' purge for horses consisted of twenty cloves of bruised garlic mixed into a pound of sweet butter which was then rolled into balls 'as big as Hen-eggs'. The consumption of five of these balls was said to be an effective means to 'work out the pestilential humours'.[54] Other 'general' or 'gentle' purges included ingredients such as senna, aloes, wormwood or rhubarb. If these proved ineffective, more 'drastic' items such as jalup, scammony or colocynth might occasionally be deemed necessary.[55]

Although such purges were suggested as an initial treatment, if they did not work readers were advised to give their animals 'clysters' [enemas] or suppositories. There were various ways in which these could be administered, from suppositories made out of butter and garlic to liquids administered through a 'clysterpipe'. The rectums of dogs and, presumably, smaller horses could also be emptied 'by means of a small hand well oiled'.[56] The treatment of large animals would have required the participation of two or more people. After rubbing the pipe and the animal's 'bellie with Oyle' it was to be inserted into his fundament, which was then to be 'stopped up' in order to keep it from falling out. In the case of a horse, the healer was supposed to 'vvalke him verie softly, and a long time, vntill that he haue voided, not onely this clyster, but vvithall some part of the dung, which he had in his bodie'.[57] Gervase Markham recommended 'thrusting a large Candle' into the fundament of the horse, pressing down its tail and holding it place in for 'a quarter of an houre, or halfe an houre'.[58] It was not, however, considered to be a

---

[53] P.T. Keyser, 'Science and Magic in Galen's Recipes' in A. Debru (ed.), *Galen on Pharmacology* (Brill, 1997), p. 178; T. Watson, *By his Majesty's Royal Letters Patent: His Instructions for the Management of Horses and Dogs* (London, 1785), p. 113 and E. Toppsell, *The Historie of Foure-Footed Beastes* (London, 1607) p 341.

[54] Anon, *The Experienced jockey, compleat horseman, or gentlemans delight* (London, 1684), p. 132.

[55] W.S.C. Copeman, *Doctors and Disease in Tudor Times* (London, 1960). p. 143.

[56] G. Markham, *A Discourse of horsmanshippe* (London, 1593), p. 45; E. Toppsell, *The Historie of Foure-Footed Beastes* (London, 1607), p 341 and T. Watson, *By his Majesty's Royal Letters Patent: His Instructions for the Management of Horses and Dogs* (London, 1785). pp. 2–3.

[57] C. Estienne, *Maison rustique,* p. 143.

[58] G. Markham, *Cheape and Good Husbandry* (London, 1614), p. 24.

good idea to treat oxen in the same manner. This may have been due to the nature of the beast and the probable difficulty of keeping the clyster in place. Instead, the reader was advised to use a smaller 'half-penny candle' and to 'put it up his Fundament as far as you can reach and leave it behind in the body'.[59]

One of the most common methods of 'physical' purging was bloodletting, or phlebotomy, which has already been discussed in the previous chapter on preventative measures. However, letting blood in a sick animal was a very different matter than carrying out the procedure on a healthy one. The use of both preventative and remedial bloodletting for animal appears much more regularly than it does for humans. One of the reasons for this may have related to the idea attributed to Pliny the Elder (23–79) who believed that wild animals practiced bloodletting for medical reasons.[60] It therefore might follow that domesticated animals would have lost that ability and would need humans to carry out the procedure for them. On the other hand, it may have been linked to the fact that one of the major decisions in undertaking phlebotomy was the strength of the patient's body and such animals were much larger and stronger than most humans. The choice of surgical instrument would depend on the type of patient. Lancets, which were regularly used on humans, were generally too flimsy to cut through fur and thicker skin. Instead, heavier instruments called 'fleams', which usually had multiple blades were used. Also, since larger creatures had much greater quantities of blood than humans, it was generally necessary to remove more in order to affect a cure.[61]

That said, phlebotomy still needed to be carried out with caution, as 'the letting of blood is very dangerous, and openeth the way to many grievous infirmities' if not properly administered. Since it was thought that properly digested food was converted into blood, starvation or death could follow the drawing of excessive amounts. It was also possible the spirits of the animal would be irrevocably depleted by the loss of too much blood. In general, it was best not to let blood when 'the signe be not in the heart, nor in the place where the incision is made'. Drawing blood 'in the day of the change of the Moone' was also not recommended, as blood levels were already thought to be low at that

---

[59] J. Lambert, *Country-man's treasure* (1676), p. 42.
[60] L. Magner, *A History of Medicine* (New York, 1992). p. 190.
[61] T.E. Crowl, 'Bloodletting in Veterinary Medicine', *Veterinary Heritage*, 19 (1996), 13–19.

time. Considerations about the movement of the planets also had to be taken into account. In general, the best time to bleed young animals was during the phase of the moon which corresponded to their age. For young animals, this was 'at the first quarter of the moon', while older ones were to be let blood in the last quarter.[62]

Many texts provided guidelines as to what part of the animal blood should be let from for specific illnesses. If a horse was suffering from 'watering eyes', it was necessary to let blood from 'his temple vaine, or the vaine under the eye'.[63] In astrological terms, the head was linked to Aries, as was the month of April. Therefore, it would have been inadvisable to carry out this procedure during that time of year. Ashwell also stressed the need to be frugal with the quantities bled:

> where the Blood is naught and most distempered, there is greatest danger of all in effusion; contrary to the opinion of some vaine Chirurgions, and idle brain'd People, who thinke that if the Blood be evil a larger quantity may be more safely exhausted.[64]

A recent archaeological find in Bath has shown that the second most common physical treatment for removing excess humours from humans was also used for animals.[65] This refers the use of various water treatments which removed impurities by forcing them through the pores in the form of sweat, which could then be wiped or washed away. Although 'artificial' sweat could also be induced through the ingestion of drugs called 'sudorificks', medicinal bathing became increasingly popular in early modern England.[66] This could take place either in a 'Naturall bath' such as a spring or in one of the many spas throughout Britain. Another option was to visit 'Artificiall baths' based on what are now called saunas or steam rooms, a concept which can be traced back to the ancient Romans 'vapporary'.[67]

The second type of therapeutic bathing was called 'waterish' and referred to the immersion of either part or the entire body of the patient

---

[62] T. Buckminster, *A newe almanacke and prognostication* (London,1589), sig. B2r; Pond, *Almanack* (Cambridge, 1641), sig. C5v; Anon., *The Gentleman's Jockey*, p. 46; S. Ashwell, *A New Almanacke and Prognostication* (London, 1641), sig. B6r and J. Lambert, *The country-man's treasure* (London, 1703), p. 59.

[63] L.W.C. *The Honest and Plaine-dealing Farrier or a Present Remedy for curing Diseases and Hurts in Horses* (London, 1636), sig. A3r.

[64] G. Naworth, *A New Almanack and Prognostication* (Oxford, 1645), sig. C3v.

[65] *Bath and North East Somerset Council Monument Full Report* (21 January 2008).

[66] N. Culpeper, *The Expert Doctors Dispensatory* (London, 1657) p. 375.

[67] Ibid, p. 197.

in water. Helmontian theory held that the water had healing properties because of the minerals and salts it acquired as it percolated through rocks and 'subterrainiean mynes.'[68] As these virtues differed according to location, spas became known for the benefits of their particular waters, although users were warned that 'Euerie medicinall water doth not cure euery infirmitie, nor everie man is to use euerie bathe.'[69] During the seventeenth century the best known spas were at Bath and Tunbridge Wells, although Scarborough, Harrogate and Buxton also catered for the ill. Wiltshire also boasted 'several Springs of the Nature and Virtue of Tunbridge-Water, some stronger, some weaker.'[70]

The spa waters in various parts of the country, and abroad, differed greatly in their mineral contents and, therefore, the types of illnesses that they were best at treating. 'Sulphur-baths', which could be found in West Yorkshire were believed to be effective therapy for 'nervous maladies, cramps, convulsions [and] palsies'. Tunbridge Wells boasted water rich in iron, which were said to 'open all manner of obstructions wheresoever they be lurking.[71] There were five main baths in Bath between the late sixteenth and the early eighteenth centuries. The waters were said to be:

> hot, of a blueish Colour, strong scent, and send forth thin Vapours; and as, without question, they have strengthened many weak and feeble Limbs, so do they cure divers Diseases by causing men to sweat either more or less proportionally to their Distempers.[72]

The biggest was known as the King's Bath, followed by the Queen's Bath, the Hot Bath, the Cross Bath and the Horse Bath. Of these, the King's Bath, Hot Bath and the Cross Bath were fed directly by springs. The King's Bath supplied the adjoining Queen's Bath with pumped water, while its refuse water was piped to the Horse's Bath which lay

---

[68] E. Jorden, *A discourse of naturall Bathes and Mineral Waters* (London, 1633), p. 8.

[69] N.G. Coley, 'Cures without Care. Chymical Physicians and Mineral Waters in Seventeenth-Century English Medicine', *Medical History*, 23 (1979), pp. 198–9 and W. Baley, *A briefe discourse of certain bathes or medicinall waters in the Countie of Warwicke* (London, 1587), sig. A3v.

[70] P. Borsay, *The English Urban Renaissance: Culture and Society in the Provincial Town 1660–1770* (Oxford, 1989), p. 32; C.F. Mullett, 'Public Baths and Health in England, Sixteenth to Eighteenth Century', *Supplement to the Bulletin of the History of Medicine* (Baltimore, 1946), p. 24 and Nicholas Culpeper, *Medicaments for the Poor*, p. 15.

[71] W. Simpson, *A Discourse of the Sulphur-bath at Knarsbrough in York-shire* (London, 1675), p. 26 and R. Rowzee, *The Queens Wells* (London, 1632), pp. 35 and 49.

[72] J. Brome, *Travels over England, Scotland and Wales* (London, 1700), pp. 38–39.

just outside the southern gate of the city.[73] The bath for horses was built 'in a Garden upon the South Side of St Jame's Church' and was used said to be effectual 'for the cure of lame and foundred horses, and the removal of some other Distempers, which are incident to those kind of Animals'.[74]

Although there was some debate as the effectiveness of drinking water from the mineral springs, it was generally agreed that this could be beneficial to one's health.[75] One contemporary source notes these healing powers on a sick horse. According to the observer, the Coachman fed his horse water from Bath over a period of six weeks. During that that time the horse 'fed and work'd as usually, and so continued for some years'.[76]

'Chyrugical' or Surgical Treatments

Nancy Siraisi has argued that the 'physical realities and technical limitations' determined both what types of conditions could be surgically treated as well as the procedures used.[77] While the former might hold true, there were a number of technological 'advances' made during this period, often on battlefields. In the sixteenth century, for example, Ambroise Paré discovered that hot oil was a particularly effective treatment for bullet wounds in both humans and animals.[78] The military surgeon William Gibson (c 1680–1750) used the knowledge he accumulated during battles to treat horses in London for almost 30 years.

On the other hand, periods of warfare also led to the spread of animal diseases. The external form of glanders, for example, manifested itself as nodules, pustules and ulcers on the skin of horses. Farcy was considered to be a highly contagious disease which could quickly spread to other types of animals. It was believed to operate by causing an 'overabundance

---

[73] J. Childrey, *Britannia Baconica, or, the Natural Rarieties of England, Scotland and Wales* (London, 1668), p. 32; and J. Wood, *An Essay towards a description of Bath* (London, 1749), p. 207.

[74] J. Wood, *An Essay towards a description of Bath* (London, 1749), p. 207 and J. Brome, *Travels*, p. 40.

[75] N. Culpeper, *Expert Doctors*, pp. 197–9.

[76] N. Salmon, *A New survey of England* (1731) Vol 1, p 810–11.

[77] N. Siraisi, *Medieval and Early Modern Medicine*, p. 154.

[78] D. Karasszon, *A Concise History of Veterinary Medicine* (Budapest, 1988), pp. 242–3 and R. Dunlop and D. Williams, *Veterinary Medicine: An Illustrated History* (London, 1996), p. 270.

of blood' which meant that sick animals needed to be bled 'on both sides of the Neck'. After this was completed the 'outward sores' were to be covered with a mixture of 'oyle of Terpentine' and 'oyle of Petre'.[79]

Another common treatment applied by laypeople was for warts or other small growths. The most benign sounding remedy for warts was to apply 'black water that stands in the root of a hollow Elm-tree'. Another suggestion for dealing with 'this Disease ... most incident of young Beasts advised tying eight or ten horsehairs tightly around the wart and leaving them until it fell off. Alternatively, it could be seared off with a hot iron, or it could be eaten away with mercury.[80]

Although more minor problems might be treated by an owner or other caretaker, most external injuries or disorders appear to have been left to specialists such as farriers or leeches. The most common surgical treatment on animals was probably that of castration which was thought to produce animals less prone to disease. It was also thought that neutering would make them easier to handle as well as producing better tasting meat.[81] Interestingly, popular medical books did not provide information on carrying out the operation itself, which was done by either ligature or cauterising, but on the precautions that readers needed to take or at what time of year it should take place. The most important concern was choosing a time when the moon was in an aspect favourable to such surgery. In general, readers were recommended to 'lib and geld' animals while the moon was in Aries, Sagittarius or Capricorn, with the most auspicious time during a lunar eclipse, or full moon.[82]

Conclusion

Although the importance of trying to provide their animals with a healthy lifestyle was widely stressed in popular medical texts it was clear that illness would eventually strike. When this occurred, it was up

---

[79] J. Brian Derbyshire, 'The eradication of glanders in Canada', in the *Canadian Veterinary Journal*, 43, 9 (September 2002), 722–726 and J. Ponteus, *The queens cabinet newly opened* (London, 1662) sig. B4v.

[80] J. Bucknall, *An Almanack* (London, 1675), sig. C2v; W. Dade, *Country-mans Almanack* (London, 1692) and 1694, sig. B1v and W. Salmon, *The London Almanac* (London, 1699), sig. B8r.

[81] K. Thomas, *Man and the Natural World* (London, 1983), p. 93.

[82] A. Clifford, *An almanack* (London, 1642), sig. C3r and Swallow, *Almanack* (Cambridge, 1646), sig. B8r.

to humans to diagnose and treat the problem. Symptoms such as list-lessness, loss of appetite or low energy would likely to have been noticed immediately given the close proximity of humans and their charges. Many texts also provided guidelines on how to determine what the dis-order was in various types of animals. This might include information on examining urine or faeces, as well as guidelines on different forms of unusual behaviour.

Once the illness was diagnosed, it was again up to humans to deter-mine whether the animal required 'a putting to' or 'a taking away of such things as are wanting, or abounding' in the body.[83] As with pre-ventative medicine, the 'dieting of the body' lay at the heart of remedial treatments with the correct type depending on the nature of the illness and the constitution of the patient. Although not as complicated as diets for sick humans, many texts provided basic dietary advice for sick animals. This included information about the qualities and natures of different types of food and drink, with suggestions about what illnesses they were good for treating. In most cases, it was recommended that the correct type of diet be supplemented with medicines meant to be retained within the body to correct humoural imbalances. These could be taken either in the form of 'simples', which contained only one ingre-dient or in more complex recipes.

As Andrew Wear has pointed out, the explanations for why remedies worked could be easily found in the popular press.[84] However, it seems likely that people were more concerned about whether something worked, rather than the reasons that lay behind it. The majority of remedies found in contemporary books were based on Galenic ideas and ingredients. In general, these encompassed mainly organic materi-als. That said, as the period covered in this book progressed it became increasingly common to include Paracelsian ingredients such as sul-phur and mercury were often included in otherwise Galenic remedies.

While the ingestion of chemicals such as mercury could be danger-ous, 'taking away' substances from the body carried greater potential dangers. This was particularly true in the case of bleeding, which may explain why texts provided so many warnings. Most other methods of purging, with the exception of going to the baths or taking the waters,

---

[83] R. Allestree, *An Almanack* (London, 1640), sig. C5r.
[84] A. Wear, *Knowledge & Practice in English Medicine* (Cambridge, 2000), p. 103.

could be carried out at home. Many authors provided instructions on how to induce vomiting, increase the flow of urine and cleanse the bowels. However, all shied away from instructing readers how to draw blood. Although such treatments were meant to rid the body of dangerous substances, they could also 'stirre the humours so violently by their nauseousnesse, that their operation is a sicknesse of it self all the while'.[85] There is also very little information on how to carry out other surgical procedures.

The type of remedial advice offered in popular medical texts showed very few changes during the early modern period. As with other types of medical information, most authors promoted an orthodox system of Galenic ingredients and theories. Although there were a handful of writers who appeared to support Paracelsian ideas, few actively promoted such ideas in these publications. As discussed in Chapter 4, there could be a variety of reasons for this. This included reassuring readers that all the material could be vouched for, generally both through their own practice and by the authors of the texts who were quoted or referred to in their own book. Alternatively, it could have been that the target audience for these works were not thought to be interested in 'new-fangled' ideas, but wanted material that would support and expand their existing knowledge.

---

[85] W. Rumsey, *Organon salutis: An instrument to cleanse the stomach* (London, 1659), sig. B2r.

EPILOGUE: VETERINARY MEDICINE IN THE EIGHTEENTH CENTURY

The previous chapters have explored various aspects of early modern veterinary medicine in England, an area that has been sadly ignored by academics. Although this facet of history is slowly gaining more serious attention by British researchers working in the modern period, the medical beliefs and practices of the early modern period are still relatively unexplored. This is partially due to the mistaken belief that a system of veterinary medicine simply did not exist in England before the late eighteenth century.[1] It might also be linked to the mystique of a dramatic growth in what might be called 'the modernisation of British society and culture'. This included medicine taking 'a move towards centre-stage' as well as developments in agriculture, commerce, communications, consumption and transport. Although the once fashionable term 'scientific revolution' is now rarely used, the period is also still lauded for developments in chemistry, mechanics and experimental philosophy.[2] As this book has previously discussed, the late eighteenth century is also credited with the beginning of a 'real' interest in animal health triggered by reoccurring episodes of 'cattle plague'. In England, the culmination of these concerns was said to be the foundation of the first London Veterinary College in 1791.[3]

---

[1] E. Cotchin, *The Royal Veterinary College: A Bicentary History* (Buckingham, 1990), p. 13; R. Dunlop and D. Williams, *Veterinary History* (London, 1996); D. Karasszon, *A Concise History of Veterinary Medicine*, trans. E. Farkas (Budapest, 1988); I. Pattison, *The British Veterinary Profession 1791–1948* (London, 1984); L. Pugh, *From Farriery to Veterinary Medicine 1785–1795* (Cambridge, 1962); F.J. Smithcors, *Evolution of the Veterinary Art: A Narrative Account to 1850* (London, 1958) and L. Wilkinson, *Animals and Disease: An Introduction to the History of Comparative Medicine* (Cambridge, 1992).

[2] R. Porter, *Bodies Politic: Disease, Death and Doctors in Britain, 1650–1900* (London, 2001), p. 31 and M. Harrison, *Disease and the Modern World: 1500 to the present* (Cambridge, 2004), p. 49.

[3] E. Cotchin, *Veterinary College*, p. 13; I. Pattison, *Veterinary Profession*, p. 1; L Pugh, 'From Farriery to Veterinary Medicine', *Veterinary History*, 75 (1975), p. 11; R. Dunlop and D. Williams, *Veterinary*, p. 266 and D. Karasszon, *Concise History of Veterinary Medicine*, p. 270.

The commonplace that what we now refer to as 'rinderpest' was the catalyst for the foundation of 'scientific' veterinary medicine in England is, however, open to debate. This is not to suggest that the disease and death of large numbers of economically valuable animals did not have a major impact on the course of history. One mid-twentieth century historian, in fact, argued that it resulted in a 'whole social and economic dislocation' in England. Inherent in this description are a range of political implications and the link with the growth of medical developments such as inoculation.[4] However, such changes do not provide sufficient evidence to credit cattle-plague with the so called metamorphosis of veterinary medicine.[5] As this book has argued, veterinary medicine at the end of the eighteenth century was little changed from a hundred years before. In the second place, the London College opened almost a century after the first outbreaks of cattle plague in England. Thirdly, the sporadic efforts to improve veterinary care in this country did not include cattle but focused exclusively on horses. Finally, the institution that was founded in the 1790's was also based entirely on treating horses, rather than the more lowly animals actually effected by the 'plague'.

As Chapter 3 has shown, there was a very real 'medical marketplace' for animals throughout the early modern period. This is hardly surprising due to the immense economic significance of working animals. Furthermore, as John Burnham has noted, in every society during all time periods 'someone plays the role of healer'. For most medical historians, however, people who treated humans are considered more worthy of serious study than those who worked with animals.[6] The continuing strength of anthropocentrism in modern society also undoubtedly contributes to the lack of attention paid to the history of animal health and illness. There is also the on-going danger of applying modern ideas and standards to the past. The fact that our modern system consists of a highly regulated and formally educated group of veterinary practitioners

---

[4] C.F. Mullet, 'The Cattle Distemper in Mid-Eighteenth-Century England', *Agricultural History*, Vol. 20, No. 3 (Jul., 1946), pp. 144–165; Dunlop and Williams, *Veterinary*, p. 291 and L. Wilkinson, *Animals & Disease*, p. 36.

[5] Readers should note that this chapter focuses exclusively on England, which experienced both a different pattern of cattle plague as well as responses to the disease than countries in Continental Europe.

[6] J.C. Burnham, *What is Medical History* (Cambridge, 2005), p. 3 and R. Porter, 'Man, Animals and Medicine at the Time of the Founding of the Royal Veterinary College' in A.R. Mitchell (ed.) *History of the Healing Professions*, Vol. III (London, 1993), p. 19.

does not negate the validity of other types of structures or types of learning. As Michael Neve has pointed out, 'it would be quite wrong and even insulting' to assume that Western medicine is more advanced or better than systems in other parts of the world'.[7]

As the previous chapters have shown, there is ample surviving evidence of a range of medical options for animals, stocked with 'professional' and lay healers offering a range of preventative and remedial measures. These illustrate the strong sense of continuity both in the veterinary advice that was disseminated through the popular press and in contemporary practices throughout the sixteenth and seventeenth centuries. While there clearly were many 'advances' in the eighteenth century, the majority appear to have little effect on the everyday system of care provided to animals in England. The dramatic growth of hospitals, for example, and the health advice that they disseminated focused exclusively on humans.[8]

There are also few signs to support the claim that 'the quantitative and objective medical system attributed to the late seventeenth and early eighteenth centuries' changed veterinary ideas or practices. Nor is there any evidence in contemporary literature that the scientific 'advances' attributed to Bacon, Descartes or the Royal Society applied to veterinary medicine.[9] That said, there were some more material changes illustrated by the occasional use of new terminology in contemporary texts. However, as many historians have noted in studies of human medicine, while physicians may have learned new ways to describe 'the body and its activities', they continued to use 'centuries-old' remedies and treatments.[10] There were some exceptions, however, possibly linked to the increased 'flow of ideas' from Continental Europe.

---

[7] J. Lane, 'Farriers in Georgian England' in A.R. Michell (ed) *The Advancement of Veterinary* Science, Vol 3 (Wallingford, 1993), 99–118 and M. Neve, 'Conclusion' in L.Conrad, M. Neve, V. Nutton, R. Porter and A. Wear (eds) *The Western Medical Tradition 800 BC to AD 1800* (Cambridge, 1996), pp. 477–494; 480.

[8] R. Porter, 'Cleaning up the Great Wen: Public Health in Eighteenth Century London', *Medical History*, Supplement No. 11, 1991: 61–75.

[9] A. Wear, 'Medical Practice in Late Seventeenth- and Early Eighteenth-Century England: Continuity and Union' in R. French and A. Wear (eds.) *The Medical Revolution of the Seventeenth Century* (Cambridge, 1989), pp. 294–5 and R. Porter, *Doctor of Society: Thomas Beddoes and the Sick Trade in Late Enlightenment England* (London, 1992), p. 23.

[10] S. De Renzi, 'Old and New Models of the Body' in P. Elmer (ed) *The Healing Arts: Health, Disease and Society in Europe 1500–1800* (Manchester, 2004), pp. 166–192.

This holds particularly true with the growth in comparative studies on human smallpox and cattle plague, which will be discussed later in this chapter.

In terms of veterinary medicine, the most dramatic historical events were linked to the formation of the first educational institutes for the teaching of veterinary medicine. London was towards the end of a queue of cities which formed schools on the Continent, with the first opening its doors in France during the early 1760's. A number of similar institutions opened up throughout Europe during the following two centuries. This raises the question of why England took so many years to follow these examples. In hindsight it seems clear that the London school made very little impact on either popular veterinary beliefs or practices. However, I would argue that it is still important as being the first formal teaching institution for animal health care, thereby beginning a trend which eventually would lead to a State sanctioned, formally licensed and regulated profession.

This chapter will examine the reasons that are normally given as being the catalyst for the development of the London College. The first is what is referred to as the 'cattle plague', a disease which decimated large herds of cattle throughout Europe in the eighteenth century. On the Continent, this triggered the involvement of government in confining and stopping its spread through mass destruction of animals. Although not ignored by the Crown, the major interventions in England came from various private individuals and groups. The types of people involved in these efforts, as well as the actual methods carried out on animals will be discussed in the second section. This is followed by the growing interest in public health and the improvement of the economy, which led to the growth of agricultural societies, who are credited with an interest in improving veterinary science. It is, of course, impossible to categorically state that none of these played a role in the eventual institutionalization of veterinary medicine. However, my research suggests that the actual catalyst and driving force behind the college was an individual blessed with imagination, drive and determination. Of course, Charles vial de St Bel (or Sainbel as he was commonly referred to in England) neither lived nor operated in a vacuum and it must be remembered that he was a product of the society and times in which he lived. He also seems to have been in the right place at the right time and managed to be introduced to the men who could make his dream of starting a veterinary college come true.

Veterinary Medicine in the Early Eighteenth Century

The medical marketplace for humans and animals at the beginning of the eighteenth century was almost identical to that of a hundred or even two hundred years before. Popular medical beliefs were still based on ancient Galenic principles, as were remedial treatments and therapies. The basic structure of healers was also unchanged, with a similar hierarchy of 'professional' and lay practitioners treating either humans and/or animals. Members of the Company of Farriers, for example, continued to be expected to serve a seven year apprenticeship in common with surgeons. Although these men have been described as 'uneducated and their ignorance was notorious', it is difficult to believe this was the general, contemporary view.[11] After all, although a relatively small number of men obtained a medical education at university, apprenticeship was still the most typical form of medical training. These were joined by a growing number of private anatomy schools starting in the 1720's with lectures on anatomy, practical physic, materia medica and chemistry. As time went on, hospitals also became sites of learning, with lecturers illustrating their lessons with clinical case studies.[12] That said, these institutions would have influenced a fairly small number of practitioners in human medicine and were no more the centre of 'professional' training than were universities.

There were also a vast range of vernacular medical books that could be used by 'professional' or lay animal healers. A large number of these 'self-help' books were attributed to the same (long-dead) authors popular in previous centuries. One of the most read authors in the early eighteenth century was Gervase Markham, who died in 1637. *Markham's Maister-piece* appeared in its sixteenth edition in 1703 with new copies coming out through the 1730's. In marketing terms, 'Gervase Markham' had become a brand name, something which it seems likely that few readers realised. Eighteenth century editions continued to provide prefaces supposedly written by Markham stating that 'I have been 50 years a Practitioner' and that his secrets were only being divulged because of 'Old-Age growing upon me'.[13] Markham's 'secrets'

---

[11] SA Hall, 'The State of the Art of Farriery in 1791', *Veterinary History*, New Series 7, 1 (January 1992), pp. 10–14.

[12] R. Porter, *The Greatest Benefit to Mankind* (London, 1997), pp. 291–293.

[13] G. Markham, *Markham's Maister-piece* (London, 1723 and 1734), sig. A2r.

were, of course, based on the ancient Greek humoural theory, as were those provided by other long-lived texts. This is illustrated by works such as *The Gentleman's Jockey and Approved Farrier* which warned in the eighth edition (1704) against treatments resulting in 'the hasty stirring up of humours in the body, where they superabound [sic] and are generally dispersed and not settled'.[14]

Jacques de Solleysel, 'querry to the French King', was another contemporary author popular over a very long period of time. The 1696 English version was a condensed version of the original French which reminded readers that although:

> We are generally so much perswaded of the Excellency of our old Writers, such as Blundevil, Markham, De la Gray, and some others, that we image none can outstrip or exceed them ... we must still acknowledge that we are in a great measure beholden to the French, for our chiefest Knowledge and Skill in this Science.[15]

In 1722 William Gibson condemned Solleysel for merely collecting earlier writings, albeit from 'the best Authors of Physick and Surgery'. This was, of course, a familiar criticism repeatedly made by seventeenth century authors Thomas Grymes, Thomas De Grey and Robert Barrett who also could have been accused of being 'mere compilers'.[16] Therefore, although certain writers may have argued that they were disseminating 'new' advice, in reality they were providing time-honoured information that their readers would been familiar and comfortable with.

Cattle Plague

Calvin Schwabe has suggested that the continuing outbreaks of 'cattle plague' in the eighteenth century marked one of the five main stages in the management of animal disease. The first focused on 'local activities', beginning in prehistoric times and lasting until the first century A.D. This was followed by a growing emphasis on military needs, which relied heavily on animal power. As a result, it was accompanied by the

---

[14] J.H. *The gentleman's jockey and approved farrier* (London, 1704), p. 2.

[15] J. de Solleysel, *The compleat horseman*, (trans.) W. Hope (London, 1692), sig. B2r.

[16] W. Gibson, *The farrier's new guide* (London, 1722), sig. A3r; T. Grymes, *The Honest and Plaine-deaing Farrier or a Present Remedy for curing Diseases and Hurts in Horses* (London, 1636), sig. A2r; T. De Grey, *The Compleat Horse-man and Expert Farrier* (London, 1651), p. 61 and R. Barrett, *The Perfect and Experienced Farrier* (London: 1660), sig. A2r.

requirement for larger scale management which lead to the development of 'basic techniques of clinical diagnoses. According to Schwabe,
this second phase ran into the early eighteenth century when it was
replaced by new requirements linked to the growth of rinderpest
epidemics. In order to combat these outbreaks, a 'Veterinary Sanitary
Police' was formed which was the major focus of the third period which
continued until about 1883.[17]

Unfortunately, there are some major problems with Schwabe's categorisations, based on what he has omitted. The importance of healthy animals
in war, for example, cannot be relegated to a particular time period. Horses,
in particular, played a key role in Western European fighting up until less
than a hundred years ago. In 1917, for example, there were 368,000 British
horses and 82,000 British mules on the Western Front. While many were
actually in cavalry units, the largest number was used for transporting
goods. During World War II, these numbers were exceeded by the vast
numbers of horses employed by the German army.[18]

Secondly, although the cattle plague had a hugely negative effective on
the economy, there is no definitive proof that this 'resulted' in the formation of 'sanitary' or 'medical police'. The terms themselves are also slightly
problematic as the meaning differs from our modern understanding of
'police'. That said, there are similarities in the sense that police aim to
maintain some form of control over the population for the overall good
of society. Mark Harrison has argued that during the eighteenth century
desire to help to ensure the health of human and animals for the 'preservation, upkeep and conservation of the labour force' resulted in this
movement towards public health.[19] Inherent in this theory is the participation of national governments which resulted in some form of policies
or other developments. In his *System einer vollstätandigen medicinischen
Polizey* [*A Compete System of Medical Police*] the Austrian physician
Johann Peter Frank (1745–1821) stressed the importance of state intervention on health issues. However, England did not have such a central-
ized system to either encourage or force medical change.[20]

---

[17] C.W. Schwabe, *Veterinary Medicine and Human Health* (Baltimore, 1984). pp.
296–298.

[18] D. Edgerton, *The Shock of the Old: Technology and Global History since 1900*
(London, 2008), pp. 34–5.

[19] M. Harrison, *Disease and the Modern World: 1500 to the present* (Cambridge,
2004), p. 61.

[20] S. De Renzi, 'Policies of Health: Diseases, poverty and hospitals' in P. Elmer (ed)
The Healing Arts (Manchester, 2004), pp. 136–16 and M. Jenner, 'Environment, health
and population' in P. Elmer (ed) *The Healing Arts* (Manchester, 2004), pp. 284–314.

This meant that the impetus to reform human or animal medicine had to come from the private sphere of individuals or groups. Roy Porter argued that this included the usage of the term 'scientific' as a 'party badge' by contemporary medical authors and practitioners. This was linked to a growing knowledge of 'gross anatomy' as well as the foundation of five large general hospitals in London between 1720 and 1745 which led to the capital becoming a major centre for surgical education.[21]

Attempts to prevent and treat the eighteenth century 'cattle plague' also came mainly from concerned individuals, some of whom were medical practitioners. It should be remembered that this was not a new disease, but had been referred to as 'the most dreaded of animal contagions' since 'time immemorial'. During the sixteenth century there were three major outbreaks occurring in England in 1500, 1514 and 1517. According to the evidence in contemporary veterinary texts, there were also numerous cases of 'cattle plague' in the later part of the sixteenth and seventeenth centuries. Due to the terminology used, it is not always possible to be sure if the authors are referring to the same or simply related illnesses. However, it seems likely that the symptoms referred to by John Fitzherbert in 1523, Fracastoro in 1530 and Leonard Mascall in 1587, were due to the spread of what we now refer to as rinderpest.[22]

Although rinderpest periodically appeared across Europe during the seventeenth century, it reached epidemic proportions on the Continent in 1709. It is thought to have begun on the banks of the Don and Volga, spreading to Moscow and beyond within a year. This was a 'violent and infectious disorder' which 'destroyed so many Cows, that most of the Dairy Farmers were ruined by it'. According to one contemporary account, the plague killed 'above 26,000 cows' in Italy during 1711.[23] The disease continued to spread and after raging through Holland and France, striking London in the summer of 1714. The first signs were 'running at the Nose and a very nauseous Breath' which led to death within three or four days. As the disease moved into Middlesex and

---

[21] M. Harrison, Disease, p. 61, W.F. Bynum, *Science and the Practice of Medicine in the Nineteenth Century* (Cambridge, 1996), p. 5 and R. Porter, 'The Eighteenth Century' in Conrad, Neve, Nutton, Porter and Wear (eds) *The Western Medical Tradition 800 BC to AD 1800* (Cambridge, 1995), p. 39.

[22] C.A. Spinage, *Cattle Plague: a history* (London, 2003), pp. 3, 96–97.

[23] Spinage, *Cattle Plague*, p 104 and 'Observations in the Distemper among Cattle', *The Gentleman's Magazine*, Vol 14, Nov. 1744, p. 585.

Essex, farmers were encouraged to isolate any healthy stock after killing and burning infected animals.[24]

There were various contemporary theories as to what caused these epidemics. According to the court physician to George I, Thomas Bates, it could spread via the clothing of 'Cow keepers' which were contaminated with 'the Infectious Effluvia of the Disease'. His suggested remedy, in common with other popular veterinary texts, was to quarantine the sick animals.[25] Similar theories and advice were propounded by a group of London physicians who met in 1745 to discuss the 'Distemper' which had become 'the Subject of Conversation and general Concern'. They believed that it spread through infected cattle, as well as on the clothing of humans or the 'Hair, Furs, Fleeces &c' of horses, sheep or dogs, who were not themselves affected by the disease. However, they added that both environmental factors and the type of food the sick animals ate could accelerate their deaths.[26] Such explanations remained popular in England throughout the century, joined by the need to immediately destroy affected animals.[27]

In 1745 the cattle plague returned to Britain with a vengeance. By 1749 it was estimated that about half a million head of cattle had died in the previous year and a half. However, these were extremely small numbers when compared to the losses on the Continent which were estimated at around three million cattle between 1740 and 1748.[28] It has been estimated that around two hundred million cattle died in Continental Europe by the end of the century.[29] According to one modern historian, the reason for these deaths was that 'there were no veterinary schools and consequently no scientifically trained veterinarians'.[30] A more recent account has suggested that the high mortality rates were due to veterinary medicine being 'non-existent both in theory and practice apart from a few treatises of diseases of the horse'.[31]

---

[24] R. Bradley, *The gentleman and farmers guide for the increase and improvement of cattle* (London, 1732), pp. 192 and 193.

[25] T. Bates, 'A brief account of the contagious disease which raged among the milch cowes near London, in the year 1714', *Philosophical Transactions*, 1718, 30: 872–885, p. 884 and F. Smith, *The Early History of Veterinary Literature*, II, p. 4.

[26] *London Magazine, or, Gentleman's Monthly Intelligencer*, 1745, p. 598.

[27] J. Mills, *A Treatise on Cattle* (London, 1776), p. 249.

[28] Spinage, *Cattle Plague*, pp. 130–133.

[29] C. Huygelen, 'The Immunization of Cattle against Rinderpest in Eighteenth Century Europe', *Medical History*, 41 (1997), 182–96.

[30] B.W. Bierer, *American Veterinary History* (Privately printed: 1940) p. 4.

[31] L. Wilkinson, Rinderpest and Mainstream Infectious Disease Concepts in the Eighteenth Century, *Medical History*, (April 1984), 28(2), 129–250.

In fact, there is no contemporary evidence to support either of these suppositions. There was a great flow of ideas on how to combat cattle plague between the Continent and Britain. On the lowest level, these included suggestions for treating and attempting to stop the spread of disease. More detailed information about larger-scale European attempts was also disseminated, including how the involvement of national or local governments, military organizations or private enterprise was leading to the formation of veterinary colleges.[32]

There was also some government involvement in Britain, but this tended to be sporadic and patchy. In general, national policy lay in the hands of the Privy Council. However, the claim that they were 'forced' to 'call in physicians to investigate' the cattle plague is not strongly supported. In 1746 the Commons passed a bill concerning the rinderpest which handed responsibility back to the council. This resulted in an ordanance ordering that all affected cattle be killed. However, it was followed by debates as to whether the state had the right to make such decisions. There was also the issue of whether animal owners would actually comply with such orders.[33]

In fact, surviving contemporary literature suggests that the general public experimented with a vast range of preventative and remedial treatments linked to perceptions of how the disease actually spread. The Italian writer Bernardino Ramizzini (1656–1714) recommended the use of variolation, the common name for inoculation, which comes from the Latin 'inoculare' which means 'to graft'. His method involved drawing a woolen thread soaked in the matter from pustules taken from infected animals into the dewlap of healthy animals.[34] However, English experts such as the previously mentioned Dr Bates suggested that segregation was a sufficient means of protection for well animals. In practice, this was probably the most common and certainly simplistic recommendation.[35]

---

[32] P. Leeflang, 'An attempt to summarize and to compare' in A. Mathijsen (ed.) *The origins of veterinary schools in Europe – a comparative view* (Utrecht, 1997), p. 72.

[33] Smithcors, *Veterinary*, p. 229 and Spinage, *Cattle Plague*, pp. 250–2.

[34] S. Riedel, 'Edward Jenner and the history of smallpox and vaccination', *Proceedings* (Baylor University Medical Center) 18(1), January 2005, 21–25.

[35] D. Karasszon, *A Concise History*, pp. 295–6; T. Bates, 'Directions', *The Gentleman's Magazine*, Vol. XV (15 October 1745), p. 528 and J. Pringle, *A rational enquiry into the nature of the plague: drawn from historical remarks on those that have already happen'd* (London, 1722), p. 12.

There were also a range of traditional remedies aimed at purging the disease from the animal's bodies. One anonymous author recommended making balls 'the bigness of Eggs' out of bay berries, garlic, rue and treacle, administered in a 'pint of small ale' and more treacle. This was to be following by covering the animal with blankets and 'stirring' him to provoke copious amounts of sweat. Another called for mixing angelica, rue, soap, tar and salt into a paste to be fed to sick animals.[36] In 1757, Peter Layard agreed with such procedures, arguing that bleeding and purging were 'all good, when properly and in due time administered' but that they became 'destructive or useless in another stage of the disease'.[37]

Other types of publications also carried a range of other 'old' and 'new' information about the plague.[38] The earliest specialist journals on health were *Medical Essays and Observations* (1733–1744) followed by *Essays and Observations* (1757–1784). The earliest veterinary journal, however, was the German *Archiv fur Rossarzte and Pferdeliebhaver* which appeared from 1788–1794, followed by *The Veterinarian* in England in 1828.[39] Medical advice and information could be found in a variety of other publications such as *The Gentleman's Magazine*, which was founded in 1731, regularly contained articles about the most pressing medical issues of the day. This included information about the cattle plague, with a major focus on preventative measures. The focus was on the time-honoured methods of purging healthy cattle regularly and not keeping more than ten or twelve together in a field. Any sick animals were to be killed, buried and covered with quick-lime, with their 'house' then washed and fumigated with burning pitch, tar or wormwood. Similar advice was given in other publications, with an emphasis on the traditional methods of preserving health through a mixture of purging, proper housing and diet.[40]

---

[36] Anon, *An Excellent Recipe for the Plague or Murrain in Cattle* (London, 1737?), p. 1 and J. Ringsted, *The cattle keeper's assistant, or genuine directions for country gentlemen* (London, 1774?), p. 40.

[37] P. Layard, *An essay on the Nature, Causes, and Cure of the Contagious Distemper among the Horned Cattle in these Kingdoms*, (London, 1757), p. 3.

[38] N. Glaisyer, Readers, correspondents and communities: John Houghton's A Collection for Improvement of Husbandry and Trade (1692–1703)' in A. Shepard and P. Washington (eds.) *Communities in early modern England: Networks, place, rhetoric* (Manchester, 2000), 235–251 and *Gentleman's Magazine*, 14 Oct 1744, p. 567.

[39] F.J. Smithcors, *Evolution of the Veterinary Art: A Narrative Account to 1850* (London, 1958); R. Porter, 'The rise of medical journalism in Britain to 1800' in W. Bynum, S. Lock and R. Porter (eds) *Medical Journals and Medical Knowledge: Historical Essays* (London, 1992). p. 8.

[40] T. Bates, 'Directions recommended to be observed in the present incurable and contagious distemper among cows', *The Gentleman's Magazine*, Vol. XV (15 October

As previously mentioned, a number of modern historians have argued that the cattle plague led directly to the foundation of veterinary colleges. Lise Wilkinson has argued that the reasons that they opened on the Continent 'in rapid succession … [was] in particular response to combat the scourge of cattle plague' because the disease was taken 'more seriously' there.[41] Sponsored by Louis XV, the school in Lyons was followed four years later with a second institute at Alford near Paris sponsored by funds provided by the minister of finance, and later agriculture, Jean Baptiste Bertin. However, it seems a bit simplistic to suggest that their sole motivation was the death of oxen and cows, rather than further reaching economic and political concerns. After all, France had more regulations, statues and certificates governing medical qualifications and practices, as well as more formal medical institutions than Britain.[42] In the following years the foundation of veterinary colleges in Turin, Padua, Parma, Dresden, Hanover, Freiburg-im-Breisgau, Karlsruhe, Berlin, Munich, Vienna, Budapest, Copenhagen and Sweden were supported by royal involvement.[43] It should be stressed, however, that these institutions were primarily concerned with the care of horses, rather than the other forms of cattle who were the main victims of the plague. In addition, it should be noted that none of the colleges had any lasting effect on cattle plague, which continued to appear with the last widespread epizootic in Britain appearing in 1865.[44]

The Role of Private Groups and Individuals

The later part of the nineteenth century is often referred to as the 'great age of public health' in Britain. This is linked to the growing involvement of central government in promoting sanitary reforms and efforts to control disease. There is, however, some debate as to whether this

---

1745), p. 528 and Anon, *A Treatise of the Plague and Pestilential Fevers, with Some Useful Hints for the bettter Preservation and Cure* (London, 1751), pp. 75–77.

[41] F.J. Smithcors, *Evolution of the Veterinary Art: A Narrative Account to 1850* (London, 1958), p. 229; M. Harrison, *Disease*, p. 61 and L. Wilkinson, 129–250.

[42] W.F. Bynum, *Science and the Practice of Medicine in the Nineteenth Century* (Cambridge, 1996), p. 7 and M. Jenner, 'Environment, health and population' in P. Elmer (ed.) *The Healing Arts* (Manchester, 2004), pp. 284–314.

[43] E. Cotchin, *The Royal Veterinary College: A Bicentenary History* (Buckingham, 1990), p. 14.

[44] J. Lane, 'A Warwickshre Cattle Plague Association', *Veterinary Record*, September 1970, 312–314.

was actually an eighteenth century phenomenon linked not to government but to the efforts of private individuals or groups.[45]

This certainly appears to be the case in veterinary medicine, whereby a number of private groups and individuals were the instigators for change. The majority were probably more interested in profit than welfare, however, particularly in terms of raising crop yields. Some men such as the Earl of Egremont, the Duke of Bedford and Thomas Coke were interested in new ideas about breeding healthier and more profitable stock.[46] The major emphasis of most veterinary reformers, however, was on the health of horses, the elite members of the animal kingdom and the ones 'more worth the Notice and Regard of Mankind, than any other of the brute creatures'.[47] As well as being the most valued, they were also the most expensive animals to buy and maintain. As Chapter 3 discussed, this resulted in a large number of healers who specialized in treating them, starting with members of the Company of Farriers through self-styled 'leeches' and lay-healers.

Interestingly, the Company of Farriers does not appear to have been involved in any attempts to 'modernise' veterinary medicine in the eighteenth century. This may have been related to the declining membership in city companies linked to the perceived lessening of the economic benefits of becoming a member.[48] In 1708 they were made up of a Master, 3 Wardens, 24 Assistants and 39 on the Livery. Unlike most other companies, they also did not have their own hall, but held only six meetings per year in a tavern, which was not as desirable as having a permanent location.[49] It may well have been that the existing members felt that their priority was to raise membership, rather than focusing on 'external' matters. D.W. Wright has estimated that there about

---

[45] D. Brunton, 'Dealing with Disease in Populations: Public Health, 1830–1880' in D. Brunton (ed.) *Medicine Transformed: Health, Disease and Society in Europe 1800–1930* (Manchester, 2004), pp. 180–207 and M. Harrison, *Disease*, p. 61.

[46] M. Overton, The Diffusion of Agricultural Innovations in Early Modern England: Turnips and Clover in Norfolk and Suffolk, 1580–1740, *Transactions of the Institute of British Geographers*, New Series, Vol. 10, No. 2 (1985), pp 205–221 and P. Horn, The Contribution of the Propagandist to Eighteenth-Century Agricultural Improvement, *The Historical Journal*, Vol. 25, No. 2 (Jun., 1982), pp. 313–329.

[47] P. Edwards, *Horse and Man in Early Modern England* (London, 2007), pp. 22–23 and W. Gibson, *The farrier's new guide,* (London, 1722), sig. A2r.

[48] J.R. Kellet, The Breakdown of Guild and Corporation Control over the Handicraft and Retail Trade in London, *The Economic History Review*, New Series, Vol. 10, No. 3 (1958), pp. 381–394.

[49] E. Hatton, *A new view of London; or, an ample account of that city, in two volumes, or eight sections,* Vol 2 (London, 1708), p. 605.

70–150 farriers working in London in any one year between 1750 and 1800.[50] However, there were only six new members in the 1750's, one in 1760 and three in 1761. The success of the company's attempts to get practicing farriers to become members can be seen in the figure of seventy-four applicants in 1762.[51]

It does not appear that refusing to join the company was a detriment to a farrier looking for work. After all, there was a great demand for the services of farriers in both town and country. A number of these men also wrote books, which called for the need to improve their art. In 1758 John Reeves explained that he was simply responding to the demands of 'several gentlemen in the neighbourhood' to publish his 'just theory of Farriery' based on his many years of practice.[52] In that same year the London farrier John Wood published a work calling on the establishment of:

> an Infirmary for the Reception of those Animals [horses] in order to have all imaginable Care taken of them and their Disorders relieved with all possible Expedition.

According to an anonymous tribute, Wood was 'no ordinary Farrier' having been 'Late Groom to the King of Sardinia, and at present Groom to the Right Hon. the Earl of Rochford'. He was not only an experienced practitioner, but the author of a tremendously successful book. First published in 1757, *A new compendious treatise of farriery* had been produced on the strength of a number of subscriptions from 'generous Personages amongst the Nobility and Gentry'.[53] His five partners in this scheme included John Girdler, William Merrick, Edward Hale, John Hubbard and William Cox. All of these were farriers, although little is known beyond that William Merrick was the son of the 'serjeant and marshall farrier to His Majesty' and Hale was 'farrier to the Second Troop of Life Guards'. Their plan was to find enough subscribers to pay an initial fee of a Guinea per horse to enable them to build an infirmary. If one of these horses needed to be taken in for care, a further nine Shillings per week was due. It was also possible for one of the staff to make house-calls, for those animals suffering either from a 'slight'

---

[50] D.W. Wright, London farriers and other veterinary workers in the 18th century, *Veterinary History*, New Series, Volt 5, No 1, Summer 1987, p. 18.

[51] Guildhall Library, *MS. 5524, Register of Freemen of the Farriers' Company*, 1777.

[52] J. Reeves, *The art of farriery both in theory and practice containing the causes, symptoms, and cure of all diseases incident to horses* (London, 1758), p. 5.

[53] J. Wood, *A new compendious treatise of farriery* (London, 1757), p. xiv.

disorder or a 'violent Malady'.[54] Unfortunately, it appears that their scheme did not succeed. While Wood's *Treatise* was popular enough to go into a second edition in 1762, there is no further mention of the infirmary.[55]

A second, more ambitious proposal followed a few years later for a teaching hospital for horses. The author was also more illustrious than Wood, being none other Edward Snape, farrier to George III and to the 'Second Troop of Life'. As a member of a farriery dynasty that was said to go back two hundred years, Snape had very powerful connections with royalty and the aristocracy. His plan was to find 3,000 subscribers who would each pay one guinea in return for free treatment. According to Edward Cotchin, this was actually established in Knightsbridge in 1778, although it swiftly closed after the promised support failed to come through.[56] Unfortunately, I have been unable to find contemporary sources to confirm this claim. However, I would suggest that a possible reason for these failures was that the target audience already had their own staff and facilities for treating their sick horses. It also suggests that although the idea might initially have sounded attractive, that it failed to continue to convince the 'market leaders', or men who could have influenced their peers, of its worth. A more likely market would have been those with smaller means who did not have such resources. On the other hand, such men may not have had the disposable income available to buy such 'insurance' for their animals.

It should also be noted that the lack of any formal institutions in England did not prevent men who wanted to study veterinary medicine from doing so. As previously mentioned, a growing number of schools opened on the Continent from the 1760's on. Going across the English Channel for higher education was a pattern that had long been followed by English physicians. In the early seventeenth century, for example, out of 814 doctors, 635 had gone to university either in Oxford, Cambridge, Padua, Leiden, Basle, Caen, Montpellier or Rheims.[57] As with physicians, prospective veterinary practitioners could also travel

---

[54] J. Wood, *A Supplement to the New Compendious Treatise of Farriery* (London, 1758), pp. 84–88 sig.A1r.

[55] J. Wood, *A new compendious treatise of farriery* (London, 1762), second edition.

[56] E.A. Gray, 'John Hunter and Veterinary Medicine', Medical *History*, 1957l Jan 1 (1), 38–50; I. Pattison, *The British Veterinary Profession 1791–1948* (London, 1984). p. 2 and E. Cotchin, *The Royal Veterinary College: A Bicentenary History* (Buckingham, 1990).

[57] J. Cule, *A Doctor for the People: 200 Years of general practice in Britain* (London, 1980), p. 60.

to the Continent to study. According to John Mills, a fellow of the Royal Society, in the 1770's 'almost every nation in Europe now sends pupils to the Royal Veterinary School at Lyons'.[58]

The Odiham Society and Charles Sainbel

In the late 1780's the Odiham Agricultural Society of Hampshire decided to start a collection to enable two English students to study there.[59] Agricultural societies were very popular in the eighteenth century, with the Odiham group being one of the earliest to start. This was also the group of men who have been lauded as the founders of the first veterinary college in England. The 'standard story' is that members of the Agricultural Society of Odiham, Hampshire formed a committee to gain support, and funds, to form a college. According to Roy Porter, they were motivated by

> the desire to create properly trained, scientifically educated, diploma wielding veterinary doctors who at long last, would practice an enlightened and humane science.[60]

In fact, the emphasis of the meeting of a small group of men at the George Inn in Odiham on the 16th of May 1783 was on 'encouraging Agriculture and Industry in the said Town and its Neighbourhood'. As with many provincial areas, a large proportion of the estimated population of 1,426 worked as agricultural labourers or farmers. In common with the rest of the country, these men were also experiencing a decline in real terms in wages while average prices were rising dramatically.[61] Although the society is mainly known for their interest in veterinary medicine, it should be pointed out that their emphasis was on how to improve farming methods to result in more lucrative crops. The Odiham group offered premiums to promote good ploughing, distributed seeds for controlled experiments and arranged for demonstration of farm machinery.[62]

---

[58] J. Mills, *A Treatise on Cattle* (London, 1776), p. iii.

[59] Veterinary College, *An account of the Veterinary College* (London, 1793), p. 8.

[60] R. Porter, 'Man, Animals and Medicine at the Time of the Founding of the Royal Veterinary College' in A.R. Mitchell (ed.), *History of the Healing Professions*, 3 (London, 1993), 19–30.

[61] B. Stapleton, 'Inherited Poverty and Life-Cycle Poverty: Odiham, Hampshire, 1650-1850', *Social History*, Vol. 18, No. 3 (Oct., 1993), pp. 339–355.

[62] P. Horn, 'The Contribution of the Propagandist to Eighteenth-Century Agricultural Improvement', *The Historical Journal*, Vol. 25, No. 2 (Jun., 1982), pp. 313–329.

Books made up of various articles on agricultural matters were very popular in the later part of the eighteenth century. The minutes of the Odiham Society from 1784 appeared in one such collection containing the first reference to the 'encouraging such means as are likely to promote the study of farriery upon rational and scientific principles'. Their plan was to 'consider what means may be most likely to encourage the study of scientific farriery' and then 'open a voluntary subscription to forward such means'.[63] On the surface, this appears to be much the same scheme which both Woods and Snape failed to implement years earlier. I would argue that the reason this one succeeded was because it was not sponsored by a farrier, or group of farriers, but by an organization made up of 'gentlemen'. It was also made up of a cross-section of men, including Thomas Burgess 'an Oxford don and distinguished ecclesiastic'. Burgess was also interested in both 'the moral improvement of farm workers' and in veterinary medicine. In 1785 he proposed the idea of an institution to formally teach farriery.[64]

Despite these encouraging noises made by the Odiham Society, there was a gap of three years before the next step was taken. As mentioned above, this was the decision to raise sufficient funds to enable two Englishmen to study in Lyons. Money was not forthcoming, however, and the students were only able to go to France in the summer of 1789. This was the same time that the French veterinarian Charles St Bel came to England and began to work on a plan for starting a college there. According to his own biographical account, he chose to live in England in order to avoid the turmoil and danger of the events which led up to the French Revolution.[65]

According to his biographer, 'Mons. de Sainbel' came to the notice of 'many noblemen and gentlemen' after dissecting the body of Eclipse, said to be one of the greatest racing horses of all times.[66] After completing his proposal in 1790, St Bel sent copies to a number of societies. It appears that the Odiham was the only group that responded in a positive way, by inviting Sainbel to become 'an honorary and Corresponding Member and one of the Committee in London'. A year later a second proposal by Sainbel was accepted and the name of the

---

[63] A. Young, *Annals of agriculture, and other useful arts*, Vol. 4 (London, 1784), pp. 195–196.

[64] L. Wilkinson, *Animals & Disease*, pp. 88–9.

[65] C. Vial de Sainbel, *The Works of Charles Vial de Sainbel* (London, 1795), p. 18.

[66] Ibid, p. 7.

working committee changed to 'The Veterinary College, London'. This committee was a splinter group of the larger mass which focused on crops and since most lived in London they decided to 'detach themselves from their body [Odiham]'. The initial list of supporters included the Prince of Wales and the Duke of York, followed by over twenty pages of additional subscribers.[67]

The initial aim was to attract sufficient funds to actually acquire a building for the new college. According to their register, however, only a fairly small number of men were actually 'subscribers to the Loan'. The need to attract more paying members was made clear by the section at the back of the book which described 'A list of Bankers and other Persons appointed to receive subscriptions to the College'.[68] The committee tried various means to publicise the new college, and attract new subscribers, one of which was to place advertisements in the classified section of *The* Times. In March 1791 their notice informed the public that a new college was 'For the reformation and improvement of Farriery' was being formed in London. It went on to 'request' that 'all the Noblemen and Gentlemen may be disposed to aid this important plan' by subscribing.[69] The first general meeting was held in September in order to discuss a 'Contract proposed to be made for Ground for building of the college'.[70] This was followed in October with an announcement of the first formal lecture to be given by Professor Sainbel at 'the temporary Residence' of the college near Saint Pancras [sic] Church on the 29th of November. Another notice asked 'all Persons wishing to become Resident or Out-Pupils' to apply to the 'Committee' or to Mr St Bel.[71]

Unfortunately, there proved to be trouble ahead both for Professor St Bel and the college. On the 4th August 1793, the Professor was 'seized with a shivering fit, attended with headach [sic], and great thirst'. This proved to be the beginning of an illness that culminated in his death on the 21st of the month. As a 'mark of kindness' the board of the college granted an annuity of sixty pounds to his widow. However, the 'present precarious income of the college' meant that the offer was retracted.[72]

---

[67] Veterinary College, *An account of the Veterinary College* (London, 1793), pp 8–10 and 49–76 and C. Vial de Sainbel, *The Works*, p. 21.

[68] Veterinary College, pp. 77–79.

[69] *The Times*, 16 March, 1791, p.1, col. A.

[70] *The Times*, 20 September 1791, p. 1, col. A.

[71] *The Times*, 4 October 1791, p. 1, col. C and 4 November 1791, p. 1, col. A.

[72] C. Vial de Sainbel, *Lectures on the elements of farriery: or, the art of horse-shoeing, and on the diseases of the foot* (London, 1793), pp. 178–9.

This was, presumably, due at least in part to Sainbel's successor, the surgeon Edward Coleman, who appeared to have little background in veterinary medicine. He began by shortening the curriculum to a few months, rather than that three years originally planned. According to Lise Wilkinson, Coleman 'ran the school to nobody's advantage save his own'.[73] This meant that, unlike the Continental veterinary colleges, the London institution offered only a brief, patchy education for aspiring farriers. It was to be well into the following century before the college became truly viable and a centre for training the men who were to become known as 'veterinary surgeons'.

Conclusion

As the early chapters have shown, the way in which a society understands and treats illness has more to do with what is happening in society than in actual germs or diseases. For most of the eighteenth century popular writers continued to propound classical ideas and theories of health and illness. Owners were advised to focus on trying to maintain a state of wellness in their animals by adhering to the principles of the seven non-naturals. Recommendations for treating those who became ill were very similar, if not identical, to those found many decades before.

While relatively few modern texts discuss early modern veterinary medicine, those that do tend to date the later part of the eighteenth century as marking the 'beginning' of the modernization of medicine. The most common explanation for this are the reoccurring episodes of 'cattle plague'. There are problems, however, with such ideas. Firstly, the early years of the college were plagued with a many staffing and financial difficulties. As a result, the numbers of people who would have been influenced by it would have been tiny. The lectures given by Sainbel during his residency disseminated very traditional advice.

Secondly, the college focused exclusively on horses, animals which were not directly affected by the cattle plague. The preventative and remedial treatments that were used throughout the century were almost identical to those from the past. Most authorities agreed that the best way to contain the disease was by swiftly isolating, then killing and burying any affected animals. The myriad of 'recipes' for treating sick

---

[73] L. Wilkinson, *Animals & Disease*, p. 97.

animals, most of which were from respected, older sources generally had little impact. England was fairly lucky countries, in that the most frequent episodes occurred on the Continent. The failure to properly research and identify the disease is most clearly seen in the horrendous outbreaks Britain experienced in the 1860's.[74]

Finally, there is no evidence to suggest that any new or innovative research was being carried out in veterinary medicine that might have lent weight to the idea of 'modernisation'. Therefore, the foundation of the college would have had little effect on popular practices which, according to the evidence in popular veterinary texts, continued much the same as before. In fact, it seems highly unlikely that most people would have been aware of what was being taught or that the College would have had any effect on their practices. Popular veterinary texts from the late eighteenth century are remarkably similar to those from earlier in the period, with most continuing to quote from classical sources. Such works contain little, if any, signs of events occurring either in the scientific community or in the growing institutionalisation of medicine.

The eighteenth century did not mark the beginning of 'modern' veterinary science in the sense of a new and improved system. It did, however, provide the kernel that would eventually result in the true the institutionalization and possibly professionalisaiton of veterinary medicine. However, this movement actually affected very few people, either as practitioners, owners or the animals themselves. Despite what many modern academics would have readers believe, this did not mean that animals were left to either be tortured by healers or left to die in pain. Instead, they continued to be cared for by a range of 'professional' and lay healers whose own interest lay in trying to keep these very valuable pieces of property healthy and productive.

---

[74] Spinage, *Cattle Plague,* pp. 182–167.

BIBLIOGRAPHY

Manuscripts

Bodleian Library, Oxford
  Wood. Alm. B(6), diary in T. Gallen's almanac, 1683.
British Library, London
  Add. MS 4403, fl. 113-119b, Pell Papers, Diary in Samuel Morland's almanac, 1650.
  Add. MS 4956, William Courten (al. Charleton), Diary in R. Saunders' almanac, 1698.
  Add. MS 18,721, Sir Robert Markham, Bart. of Sedgebroke, Diary in J. Gadbury's almanac, 1681.
  Add. MS 22,550, Henry Hyde, Second Earl of Clarendon, Diary in J. Goldsmith's almanac, 1691.
Buckinghamshire Records Office, Aylesbury
  D/X 581/2, John King of Steeple Claydon, Diary in Rider's *British Merlin*, 1687.
Guildhall Library, London.
  Guildhall MS. 2890 Blacksmith's Company, Articles of Farriers by-laws submitted to Court of Aldermen in 1359, c. 17th century.
  Guildhall MS. 5534-4 Farrier Court Journals [1674–1867].
  Guildhall MS. 5526, Company of Farriers Apprentice Records, 17th/18th century.

Printed Primary Sources

A.S., *The Gentleman's Compleat Jockey: with the Perfect Horseman and Experience'd Farrier* (London, 1697).
Agrippa, Henry Cornelius, *The Vanity of Arts and Sciences* (London, 1964).
Albertus, Magnus, *On Animals: A Medieval Zoological Summary*, Vol I, Kitchell, K.F. and I.M Resnick (trans.) (Baltimore, 1999).
Allestree, Richard, *A new almanack and prognostication* (London, 1614, 1618 and 1640).
Almond, Robert, *The English Horsman and Complete Farrier* (London, 1673).
Ambrose, Paré, *The Workes* (London, 1634).
Andrews, William, *The Astrological Physitian* (London, 1656).
——, *Newes from the starres* (London, 1680).
Anonymous, *The English Farrier, or, Countrey-mans Treasure* (London, 1631).
——, *A Physical dictionary, or, An Interpretation of such crabbed words and terms of arts, as are deriv'd from the Greek or Latin, and used in physick, anatomy, chirurgery, and chymistry* (London, 1657).
——, *The Gentleman's Jockey, and Approved Farrier* (London, 1676).
——, *The Experienced Jockey, Compleat Horseman, or Gentlemans Delight* (London, 1684).
——, *An Excellent Recipe for the Plague or Murrain in Cattle* (London, 1737?).
——, *A Treatise of the Plague and Pestilential Fevers, with Some Useful Hints for the better Preservation and Cure* (London, 1751).

——, *A Brief Examination of the Views of the Veterinary College* (London, 1795).

Ashwell, Samuel, *A New Almanacke and Prognostication* (London, 1641).

Askham, Anthony, *A Litell treatyse of Astronomy, very necessary for Physyke and Surgerye* (London, 1550).

Atkinson, C., *Panterpre: or, a pleasant almanack* (London, 1673).

Ball, W, *A Briefe Treatise Concerning the Regulating of Printing* (London, 1651).

Barker, J., An *account of the present epidemical distemper amongst the black cattle* (London, 1745).

Barret, Robert, *The Perfect and Experienced Farrier* (London, 1660).

Baston, J., *Mercurius hermeticus ephemeris* (London, 1657).

Bates, Thomas, 'Directions recommended to be observed in the present incurable and contagious distemper among cows', *The Gentleman's Magazine*, Vol. XV (15 October 1745).

Beridge, F., *Ephemeris* (London, 1654).

Blagrave, Joseph, *Blagrave's Astrological Practice of Physick* (London, 1689).

——, *The Epitome of the Art of Husbandry* (London, 1670).

Blagrave, William, *Blagrave's Ephemeris* (London, 1659).

Blome, R., *The gentlemans recreation in two parts* (London, 1686).

Booker, John, *Telescopium Uranicum* (London, 1661).

Boord, Andrew, *A Compendious Regiment, or Dietarie of Health* (London, 1576).

Bowker, John, *A New Almanack* (London, 1679).

Bracken, Henry, *Farriery Improved: or, a compleat treatise upon the art of farriery* (London, 1737).

Bradley, R. *A survey of the ancient husbandry and gardening* (London, 1725).

Buckminster, Thomas, A *newe almanacke and prognostication* (London, 1589).

Bucknall, John, *Calendarium Pastoris or The Shepherds* [sic] almanack (London, 1675 and 1676).

Burton, R. *Anatomy of Melancholy* (London, 1621).

C.H., B.C., C.M., Ingenious Artists, *The Perfect Husbandman, or The Art of Husbandry* (London, 1657).

Caius, J., *Of English Dogges* (London, 1576).

City and Countrey Chapmans Almanack, (London, 1687).

Claridge, John, *The Shepheard's Legacy* (London, 1670).

Clarke, R., *Clark an almanack* (London, 1634).

Clarke, William, A *new almanacke* (London, 1668).

Clifford, Arthur, *An almanack* (London, 1642).

Clifford, Christopher, *The schoole of horsemanship* (London, 1585).

Cocke, Thomas, *Kitchin-Physick: or, Advice to the Poor, By Way of Dialogue* (London, 1676).

Coelson, Lancelot, *An almanack* (London, 1680).

——, *Nuncious Coelestis* (London, 1676).

——, *The poor-mans physician and chyrugion* (London, 1656).

Cogan, Thomas, *The Haven of Health* (London, 1612).

Colbatch, John, *Four Treatises of Physick and Chirurgery* (London, 1698).

Cox, N., *The gentleman's recreation: in four parts* (London, 1697).

Crankanthorp, John, *Accounts of the Reverend John Crankanthorp of Fowlmere 1682–1710*, eds. Paul Brassley, Anthony Lambert and Philip Saunders (Cambridge, 1988).

Crawshey, John, *The Countrymans Instructor* (London, 1636).

Crowshey, John, *The Good-husbands Jewel* (Yorke, 1661).

Culpeper, Nicholas, *The English Physitian, or an Astrolog-Physical Discussion of the Vulgar Herbs of this Nation* (London, 1652).

——, *Culpeper's Complete Herbal and English Physician Enlarged* (London, 1653, reprint Ware, 1995).

——, *Pharmacopoeia Londinensis: or the London Dispensatory* (London, 1653).

——, *New Method of Physick* (London, 1654).

——, *Galen's Art of Physick* (London, 1657).

——, *The Expert Doctor Dispensatory* (London, 1657).

——, *Astrological Judgement of Diseases* (London, 1665).

——, *Culpeper's School of Physick* (London, 1678).

——, *Semeiotica Uranica, or an Astrological Judgment of Disease* (London, 1651).

Dade, William, *The Country-mans Kalendar* (London, 1684 and 1700).

Dariot, Claude, *A briefe and most easie introduction to the astrologicall judgment of the starres* (London, 1598).

DeGrey, Thomas, *The Compelat Horse-man and Expert Ferrier* (London, 1651).

De Henley, W., *The Boke of Husbandrie.* (London, 1503).

Dixon, Roger, *Consultum Sanitatis, A Directory to Health, Displayed in Several Choice Medicines* (London, 1663).

Dove, *An almanack* (London, 1638).

Dubrauius, Ianus, *A new book of good husbandry* (London, 1599).

E.R., *The Experienced Farrier, or, Farring Completed* (London, 1678).

Elyot, Thomas, *The Castel of Helthe* (London, 1539).

Estienne, C., *Maison rustique, or The countrey farme* (London, 1616).

Evans, J., Almanack (London, 1629).

Fitzherbert, John, *The Booke of Husbandry* (London, 1573).

Fowle, Thomas, Speculum *uranicum* (London, 1695).

G.L., *The Gentleman's new jockey: or, Farrier's approved guide* (London, 1691).

Gadbury, John, Thesaurus *Astrologiae* (London, 1674).

Gallen, Thomas, *An Almanack and Prognostication* (London, 1683).

Gardner, Robert, *Veterinarium Meteorologist Astrology* (London, 1698).

Gerard, John, *The herbal or Generall historie of plants* (London, 1597).

Gibson, William, *The farrier's new guide* (London, 1722).

——, *The herbal or Generall historie of plants* (ed.) T. Johnson (London, 1633).

Glaisyer, N., Readers, correspondents and communities: John Houghton's A Collection for Improvement of Husbandry and Trade (1692–1703)' in A. Shepard and P. Washington (eds.) *Communities in early modern England: Networks, place, rhetoric* (Manchester, 2000), 235-251.

Gray, E.A., 'John Hunter and Veterinary Medicine', Medical *History*, 1957l Jan 1 (1), 38–50.

Grymes, Thomas, *The Honest and Plaine-dealing Farrier or a Present Remedy for Curing Diseases and Hurts in Horses* (London, 1636).

Halfpenny, John, *The gentlemans jockey and approved farrier* (London, 1676).

Hart, J., *Klinike, or The Diet of the Diseased* (London, 1633).

Harward, Michael, *The Herds-man's Mate: Or, a Guide for Herds-men* (Dublin, 1673).

Hatton, E., *A new view of London; or, an ample account of that city, in two volumes, or eight sections*, Vol 2 (London, 1708).

Hill, Thomas, *A necessary almanack* (London, 1572).

Hippocrates, *On Ancient Medicine*, (trans) M.J. Schiefsky (Leiden, 2005).

Holden, Mary, *The Womans* [sic] *Almanack* (London, 1688).

J.B., gent., The Epitome of the Art of Husbandry (London, 1670).

Jorden, E., *A discourse of naturall Bathes and Mineral Waters* (London, 1633).

Kellet, J.R., The Breakdown of Guild and Corporation Control over the Handicraft and Retail Trade in London, *The Economic History Review*, New Series, Vol. 10, No. 3 (1958), pp. 381–394.

Lambert, J., *The Countrymans Treasure* (London, 1676).

Lambrocke, T., *Milke for children, or, A plain and easie method teaching to read and write* (London, 1685).

Langrish, B., *The Modern Theory and Practice of Physic. Wherein The Antecedent Causes of Diseases; The Rise of the most Usual Symptoms incident to them; And the True Methods of Cure* (London, 1635).

Layard, P., *An essay on the Nature, Causes, and Cure of the Contagious Distemper among the Horned Cattle in these Kingdoms*, (London, 1757).

LeClerc, Daniel, *The History of Physick, or an Account of the Rise and Progress of the Art* (London, 1699).

Lilly, William, *Christian Astrology* (London, 1647).

——, *Merlinus Anglicus Junior* (London, 1644).

Lovell, W., *The Dukes desk newly broken up: Wherein is discovered Divers Rare Receipts of Physick and Surgery* (London, 1661).

L.W.C., *The English Farrier, Or, Country-mans treasure* (London, 1639).

——, *The Honest and Plaine-dealing Farrier or a Present Remedy for curing Diseases and Hurts in Horses* (London, 1636).

Manning, J., *A new booke, intituled, I am for you all, complexions castle* (London, 1604).

Markham, Gervase, *Markham's Maister-piece* (London, 1615, 1636, 1683, 1703, 1723 and 1734).

——, *Markham's Master-piece Revived* (London, 1681).

——, *A Way to Get Wealth* (London, 1661).

——, *Markham's Faithfull Farrier* (London, 1638).

——, *Cheape and Good Husbandry* (London, 1616).

——, *The English Housewife*, ed. Michael Best (London, 1615, reprint London, 1986).

——, *Countrey Contentments* (London, 1615).

——, *Cavelrice, Or The English Horseman: Contayning all the Arte of Horse-manship* (London, 1607).

——, *A Discourse of horsmanshippe* (London, 1593).

Mascal, Leonard, *The first booke of cattell* (London, 1587).

——, *The Government of Cattle* (London, 1662).

——, *The husbandlye ordring and gouernmente of poultrie* (London, 1585).

Maynwaringe, E., *The method and means of enjoying health, vigour, and long life* (London, 1683).

Mills, J., *A Treatise on Cattle* (London, 1776).

More, P., *The hope of health* (London, 1565).

Mortimer, J., *The whole art of husbandry: or, the way of managing and improving of land.* (London, 1721).

Muffett, Thomas, *Healths Improvement: or, Rules Comprizing and Discovering The Nature, Method, and Manner of Preparing all sorts of Food* (London, 1655).

N.P., *The Vertue and Operation of this Balsame* (London, 1615).

Naworth, G., *A New Almanack and Prognostication* (Oxford, 1645).

Parkinson, J.,*Theatrum Botanicum: the Theatre of Plants or, an Herball of Large Extent* (London,1640).

Partridge, John, *The Widdowes Treasure Plentifully Furnished with Sundry secrets* (London, 1631).

Paynell, Thomas, *Regimen sanitatis Salerni* (London, 1539).

Peachem, Henry, *The Complete Gentleman, The Truth of our Times, and The Art of Living in London* (London, 1622).

Pelling, M. and F. White, *Medical Conflicts in Early Modern London: Patronage, Physicians, and Irregular Practioners, 1550–1640* (Oxford, 2003).

Pepys, Samuel, *The Diary of Samuel Pepys*, eds. Robert Latham and William Matthews (London, 1970-83: 11 volumes).

Percival, J., *The English Travels of Sir John Percival and William Byrd II*, (ed.) M.R. Wagner (Columbia, Missouri, 1989).

Physiologus, P. *The Good housewife made a Doctor* (London, n.d.).

Poole, John, *Country Astrology in Three Books* (London, 1650).

Poole, William, *The Country Farrier* (London, 1652).

Poor Robin, *Poor Robin's Almanack* (London, 1682).

Pringle, J., A *rational enquiry into the nature of the plague: drawn from historical remarks on those that have already happen'd* (London, 1722).

Reeves, J.,*The art of farriery both in theory and practice containing the causes, symptoms, and cure of all diseases incident to horses* (London, 1758).

Ringsted, J., The *cattle keeper's assistant, or genuine directions for country gentlemen* (London, 1774?).

Rogeford, Henry, *An Almanack* (London, 1561).

Rowze, R. *The Queens Wells* (London, 1632).

Rumsey, William, *Organon salutis: An instrument to cleanse the stomach* (London, 1659).

Sainbel, C. Vial de, *The Works of Charles Vial de Sainbel* (London, 1795).

——, *Lectures on the elements of farriery: or, the art of horse-shoeing, and on the diseases of the foot* (London, 1793).

Salmon, William, *Synopsis Medicinae: Or, a Compendium of Physick* (London, 1671).

——, *Pharmacopoeia Londinensis. Or, the New London Dispensatory* (London, 1685).

——, *The London Almanac* (London, 1697).

——, *Salmon's Family Dictionary, or Household Companion* (London, 1702).

Saunders, Richard, *The Astrological Judgment and Practice of Physick* (London, 1677).

——, *Apollo Anglicanus* (London, 1674 and 1678).

Sea-mans Almanack (London, 1655).

Smith, J., *Profit and pleasure united: or, the husbandman's magazine* (London, 1704).

Snape, Andrew, *The Anatomy of an Horse* (London, 1683).

Snape, Edward, *Snape's Practical Treatise on Farriery* (London, 1791).

Sofford, F., *A new almanack* (London, 1621).

Solleysel, S., *The Parfait Mareschal or Compleat Farrier*, trans. Sir W. Hope (Edinburgh, 1696).

Speed, Adolphus, *The gentleman's compleat jockey* (London, 1682).

Stevens, Charles and John Liebault, *Maison Rustique, Or, The Countrey Farme*, (trans.) Richard Surflet (London, 1616).

Swaine, John, Every *Farmer his own Cattle-Doctor* (London, 1786).

Swallow, *Almanack* (Cambridge, 1646).

Swan, *Ephemeris* (Cambridge, 1657).

Tanner, John, *The Hidden Treasures of the Art of Physick* (London, 1659).

——, *Angelus Britannicus* (London, 1697).

Toppsell, Edward, The *Historie of Foure-Footed Beastes* (London, 1607).

Trigge, T., *Calendarium Astrologicum* (London, 1676 and 1681).

Tryon, Thomas, *The Country-man's Companion, or A New Method of Ordering Horse & Sheep* (London, 1688).

Turner, William, *A new boke of the natures and properties of all wines that are commonly used here in England* (London, c.1568).

Tusser, Thomas, *Five Hundred Points of Good Husbandry* (London, 1553).

Vaughn, William, Directions *for Health, both Naturall and Artificiall* (London, 1617).

Vegetius, F., *The foure bookes of Flavius Renatus Vegetius* (trans.) J. Sadler (London, 1572).

Venner, T., *Via recta ad vitam longam, or, A plain philosophicall demonstration* (London, 1638).

Veterinary College, *An account of the Veterinary College* (London, 1793).

Walkington, Thomas, *The optick glasse of humors. Or The touchstone of a golden temperature, or the Philosophers stone to make a golden temper* (London, 1607).

Watson, Thomas, *Instructions for the Management of Horses and Dogs* (London, 1785).

Wing, Vincent, *An Almanac and Prognostication* (London, 1643).

Winstanley, William, The *country-man's guide or plain directions for ordering. Curing. breeding choice, use and feeding. Of horses, cows, sheep, hoggs, &c* (London, 1679).

Wood, J., *A new compendious treatise of farriery* (London, 1757).

——, *An Essay towards a description of Bath* (London, 1749).
Wood, O., *An Alphabetical Book of Physicall Secrets* (London, 1639).
Woodhouse, John, *A new almanacke and prognostication* (London, 1634).
Young, A., *Annals of agriculture, and other useful arts*, Vol. 4 (London, 1784).

Secondary Sources

Adams, A. *The History of the Worshipful Company of Blacksmiths* (London, 1951).
Adams, J.N., *Pelagonius and Latin Veterinary Terminology in the Roman Empire* (Leiden, 1995).
Ainsworth, G.C., *Introduction to the History of Medical and Veterinary Mycology* (Cambridge, 1986).
Albala, Ken, *Eating Right in the Renaissance* (Berkeley, California, 2002).
——, *Food in Early Modern Europe* (Westport, Conn., 2003).
Arnold, Ken, Roy Porter and Lise Wilkinson, *Animal Doctor – Birds and Beasts in Medical History: An Exhibition at the Wellcome Institute for the History of Medicine* (London, 1994).
Ash, E.A., *Dogs and Their History and Development* (London, 1927), Vol.II.
Baransky, A., *Geschichte der Thierzucht und Thiermedicin* (Vienna, 1886).
Barber, R. *Bestiary* (Woodbridge, 1999).
Barton, Tamsyn S., *Power and Knowledge: Astrology, Physiognomics, and Medicine under the Roman Empire* (Ann Arbor, 2002).
Bates, D.G., 'Why Not Call Modern Medicine Alternative'?, *Perspectives in Biology and Medicine*, 43.4 (2000) 502-518.
Bauer, H., *Science or Pseudoscience: Magnetic Healing, Psychic Phenomena and other Heterodoxies* (Champaign, 2001).
Beier, L.M., *Sufferers and Healers: The Experience of Illness in Seventeenth Century England* (London, 1987).
Bell, F.R., 'The Days of the Farriers', *Veterinary History*, 9 (1977), 3–6.
Bennett, H.S., *English Books and Readers 1558 to 1603* (Cambridge, 1965).
Blaisdell, John D., 'Rabies in Shakespeare's England', *Historia Medicinae Veterinariae*, 16 (1991), 1–80.
——, 'The Deadly Bite of Ancient Animals', *Veterinary History, New Series*, 8 (London, 1994), 22–27.
Broad, John, 'Cattle Plague in Eighteenth Century England' The Agricultural History Review vol. 31, no. 2 (1983), pp. 104–115.
Budiansky, S., *The Covenant of the Wild: Why Animals Chose Domestication* (New York, 1992).
Burnham, C., *What is Medical History?* (Cambridge, 2005).
Bury, Michael, *Health and Illness* (Cambridge, 2005).
Bynum, W. F., *Science and the Practice of Medicine in the Nineteenth Century* (Cambridge, 1996).
Capp, Bernard, *Astrology & the Popular Press: English Almanacs 1500-1800* (London, 1979).
Carey, Hilary M., *Courting Disaster: Astrology at the English Court and University in the Later Middle Ages* (London, 1992).
Carroll, P.E., 'Medical Police and the History of Public Health', *Medical History*, 2002, 46: 461–94.
Carter, Henry, 'The History of Rabies', *Veterinary History*, New Series, 9 (London, 1996), 20–31.
Chapman, Allan, 'Astrological Medicine' in Charles Webster (ed.) *Health, Medicine and Morality in the Sixteenth Century* (Cambridge, 1979), 275–300.

Coburn, D. and E. Willis, 'The Medical Profession: Knowledge, Power and Autonomy' in G.L. Albrecht, R. Fitzpatrick and S.C. Scrimshaw (eds) *The Handbook of Social Studies in Health & Medicine* (London, 2000), pp. 377–93.

Cockayne, O., *Leechdoms, Wortcunning and Starcraft of Early England* (London, 1865).

Cook, Harold J., 'Good Advice and Little Medicine: The Professional Authority of Early Modern English Physicians', *Journal of British Studies*, 33 (January 1994), 1–31.

——, *The Decline of the Old Medical Regime in Stuart London* (London, 1986).

Cook, Judith, *Dr. Simon Forman: A Most Notorious Physician* (London, 2001).

Corbain, A., *The Foul & The Fragrant: Odour and the Social Imagination* (London, 1996).

Cotchin, Ernest, *The Royal Veterinary College: A Bicentenary History* (Buckingham, 1990).

Cross, G., *A Social History of Leisure Since 1600* (State College, PA, 1990).

Crowl, Thomas E., 'Bloodletting in Veterinary Medicine', *Veterinary Heritage*, 19 (1996), 15–19.

Cuneo, Pia, Beauty and the Beast, *Journal of Early Modern History*, 4, no 3–4 (2000) 269–321.

Curry, Patrick, *Prophecy and Power: Astrology in Early Modern England* (Princeton, 1989).

Curth, Louise Hill, 'History of Health and Illness' in J. Naidoo and J. Wills (ed.) *Health Studies: an introduction*, 2nd edition (London, 2008), 47–72.

——, *English Almanacs, astrology and popular medicine: 1550–1700* (Manchester, 2007).

——, 'A Remedy for his Beast: animal health care in early modern Europe', *Intersections: representations of animals, Yearbook for Early Modern Studies*, 6 (2007).

——, 'Introduction: Perspectives on the Evolution of the Retailing of Pharmaceuticals' and 'Medical Advertising in the Popular Press' in L. Hill Curth (ed.) *From Physick to Pharmaceuticals: Five Hundred Years of British Drug Retailing* (Aldershot, 2006), pp. 1–12 and 29–48.

——, 'The Medical Content of English Almanacs', *Journal of the History of Medicine and Allied Sciences* (July 2005), pp. 255–282.

——, 'Astrological Medicine and the Popular Press in Early Modern England', *Cosmos and Culture*, 9, No. 1 (Spring/Summer 2005), pp. 73–94.

——, 'Animals, Almanacs and Astrology: Seventeenth Century Animal Health Care in England', *Veterinary History*, 12 (November 2003), pp. 33–54.

——, 'Almanacs as Medical Mediators' in C. Usborne and W. de Blecourt (eds) *Mediating Medicine: Cultural approaches to illness and treatment in early modern and modern England* (Routledge, 2003), pp. 56–70.

——, 'The Care of the Brute Beast: Animals and the Seventeenth-Century Medical Marketplace', *Social History of Medicine*, 15 (2002), pp. 375–392.

——, 'English Almanacs and Animal Health Care in the Seventeenth Century', *Society and Animals*, 8 (2000), pp. 71–86.

Davis, Dorothy, *A History of Shopping* (London, 1966).

Demaitre, L. 'The Art and Science of Prognostication in Early University Medicine', *Bulletin of the History of Medicine*, 77.4 (2003).

Derbyshire, B.J., 'The eradication of glanders in Canada', in the *Canadian Veterinary Journal*, 43, 9 (September 2002), 722–726.

De Renzi, S., 'Old and New Models of the Body' in P. Elmer (ed.) *The Healing Arts: Health, Disease and Society in Europe 1500–1800* (Manchester, 2004), pp. 166–192.

Dewhurst, Kenneth, *Willis' Oxford Casebook* (Oxford, 1981).

Doel, M.A. and J. Segrett, 'Self, Health, and Gender: complementary and alternative medicine in the British mass media', *Gender, Place and Culture*, 10, 2 (June 2003), 131–44.

Dolby, S.K., *Self-Help Books: Why Americans Keep Reading Them* (Champaign, 2005).

Doyen-Higuet, Anna-Marie, The 'Hippiatria' and Byzantine Medicine, *Dumbarton Oaks*, 3 (1984), 111–120.

Dunlop, Robert and David Williams, *Veterinary Medicine – An Illustrated History* (Chicago, 1996).

Edgerton, D., *The Shock of the Old: Technology and Global History since 1900* (London, 2008).

Edwards, Peter, *The Horse Trade of Tudor and Stuart England* (Cambridge, 1988).

——, *Horse and man in Early Modern England* (London, 2007).

Eisenstein, Elizabeth, *The Printing Revolution in Early Modern Europe* (Cambridge, 1983).

Fissell, Mary E., 'Readers, Texts, and Contexts: Vernacular Medical Works in Early Modern England' in Roy Porter (ed.) *The Popularization of Medicine 1650–1850* (London, 1992).

Fox, A., *Oral and Literate Culture in England 1500–1700* (Oxford, 2000).

French, Roger, Medicine *before Science: The Business of Medicine from the Middle Ages to the Enlightenment* (Cambridge, 2003).

Fudge, Erica, *Perceiving animals: humans and beasts in early modern Culture* (Basingstoke, 2000).

Furdell, Elizabeth Lane, *Publishing and Medicine in Early Modern England* (Rochester, N.Y., 2002).

Galton, F, 'The First Steps Towards the Domestication of Animals', *Transactions of the Ethnological Society of London*, N.S. 3, 122–138.

George, W. and B. Yapp, *The Naming of Beasts: Natural history in the medieval bestiary* (London, 1991).

Glanville, P., 'The City of London' in P. Glanville (ed) *The Cambridge Cultural History*, Vol.4, 17th Century Britain (Cambridge,1992).

Grafton, Anthony, 'Starry Messengers: Recent Work in the History of Western Astrology', *Perspectives on Science*, 8, No. 1 (2000), 70–83.

Grant, Mark, *Galen on Food and Diet* (London, 2000).

Gray, E.A., 'John Hunter and Veterinary Medicine', *Medical History*, 1957, (1), 38–50.

Greaves, David, *The Healing Tradition: Reviving the soul of Western Medicine* (Oxford, 2004).

Gunnarsson, S., 'The conceptualisation of health and disease in veterinary medicine', *Acta Veterinaria Scandinavica*, 2006, 48:20, 1–6.

Haas, Kenneth, Animal Therapy Over the Ages: 8. Self-Treatment', *Veterinary Heritage*, Vol. 25, No. 2 (November 2002), 37–40.

Hackel, H. Brayman, *Reading Material in Early Modern England: Print, Gender and Literacy* (Cambridge, 2005).

Hall, S. A., 'The State of the Art of Farriery in 1791', Veterinary History, New Series 7, 1 (January 1992), pp. 10–14.

Harwood, D., Love for Animals and How it Developed in Great Britain (New York, 1928.)

Harrison, Mark, *Disease and the Modern World 1500 to the present Day* (Cambridge, 2004).

——, 'From medical astrology to medical astronomy: sol-lunar and planetary theories of disease in British medicine, c. 1700–1850', *The British Journal for the History of Science*, 33 (2000), 25–48.

Harrison, Peter, 'Descartes on Animals', *The Philosophical Quarterly*, 42, No 167 (April, 1992), 219–227.

Hellinga, L. and J.B. Trapp (eds.) *The Cambridge History of the Book in Britain*, Vol. III 1400–1557 (Cambridge, 1999).

Henry, J., 'Doctors and healers: popular culture and the medical profession' in S. Pumfrey, P.L. Rossi and M. Slawinski (eds) *Science, culture and popular belief in Renaissance Europe* (Manchester, 1991), pp. 191–221.

Hirschman, E.C. 'Consumers and Their Animal Companions', *The Journal of Consumer Research*, Vol. 20, No. 4 (Mar., 1994), pp. 616–632.

Horn, Pamela, The Contribution of the Propagandist to Eighteenth-Century Agricultural Improvement, *The Historical Journal*, Vol. 25, No. 2 (Jun., 1982), pp. 313–329.

Houston, R.A., *Literacy in Early Modern Europe* (London, 1988).

Huygelen, C., 'The Immunization of Cattle against Rinderpest in Eighteenth Century Europe', *Medical History*, 41 (1997), 182–96.

Hyland, Ann, *The Horse in the Middle Ages* (Stroud, 1999).

Jankovic, V., Reading *the skies: a cultural history of English weather, 1650–1820* (Manchester, 2000).

Jenner, Mark, 'The Great Dog Massacre' in W. Naphy and P. Roberts (eds) *Fear in early modern society* (Manchester, 1997), pp. 44–61.

——, 'Environment, health and population' in P. Elmer (ed.) *The Healing Arts* (Manchester, 2004), 284–314.

Johns, Adrian, *The Nature of the Book: Print and Knowledge in the Making* (Chicago, 1998).

Jones, E.L., *Seasons and Prices: The Role of the Weather in English Agricultural History* (London, 1964).

Jones, Peter Murray, 'Medicine and Science' in Lotte Hellinga and J.B. Trapp (eds.) *The Cambridge History of the Book in Britain*, 3, 1450–1557 (Cambridge,1999), 433–49.

——, 'Image, Word, and Medicine in the Middle Ages' in J.A. Givens, K.M. Reeds, A. Touwaide (ed.) *Visualizing Medieval Medicine and Natural History, 1200–1550* (Aldershot, 2006).

Jones, Susan D., *Valuing Animals: Veterinarians and Their Patients in Modern America* (Baltimore, 2002).

Jouana, J., 'The Birth of Western Medical Art' in M. Grmek (ed) *Western Medical Thought from Antiquity to the Middle Ages* (London, 1998), pp. 22–71.

Karasszon, Denis, *A Concise History of Veterinary Medicine*, trans. E. Farkas (Budapest, 1988).

Keiser, George R., 'Medicines for Horses: A Medieval Veterinary Treatise', *Veterinary History*, New Series, Vol 12, No 2 (2004), 125–148.

Keyser, P.T., 'Science and Magic in Galen's Recipes' in A. Debru (ed.), *Galen on Pharmacology* (Leiden, 1997).

Lane, Joan, A Warwickshre Cattle Plague Association', *Veterinary Record*, September 1970, 312–314.

——, 'The Role of Apprenticeship in Eighteenth-Century Medical Education in England' in W.F. Bynum and Roy Porter (eds) *William Hunter and the Eighteenth Century Medical World* (Cambridge, 1985), 57–105.

——, 'Farriers in Georgian England' in A.R. Mitchell (ed.) *History of the Healing Professions*, 3 (Cambridge, 1993), 99–117.

——, *Apprenticeship in England 1600–1914* (London, 1996).

Leeflang, Peter, P. Leeflang, 'An attempt to summarize and to compare' in A, Mathijsen (ed.) *The origins of veterinary schools in Europe – a comparative view* (Utrecht, 1997).

Lesniak, M., Animals and The Veterinarian in Ancient Rome, *Veterinary Heritage*, Vol 20, 2 (November 1997) 45–52.

Lindemann, Mary, *Medicine and Society in Early Modern Europe* (Cambridge, 1999).

McCabe, Anne, *A Byzantine Encyclopedia of Horse Medicine: The Sources, Compilation, and Transmission of the Hippicatrica* (OUP, 2007).

McKitterick, Rosamund, 'Books and sciences before print' in R. McKitterick (ed.) *Books and the Sciences in History* (Cambridge, 2001), 13–24.

MacDonald, Michael, 'The Career of Astrological Medicine in England' in Ole Grell and Andrew Cunningham (eds) *Religio Medici – Medicine and Religion in Seventeenth Century England* (Aldershot, 1996), 62–90.

Maehle, Andreas-Holger and Ulrich Tröhler, 'The Ethical Discourse on Animal Experimentation, 1650–1900' in Andrew Wear, Johanna Geyer-Kordesch and Roger French (eds) *Doctors and Ethics: The Earlier Historical Setting of Professional Ethics* (Amsterdam, 1993), 203–51.

——, 'Animal Experimentation from Antiquity to the End of the Eighteenth Century: Attitudes and Arguments' in N.A. Rupke (ed.) *Vivisection in Historical Perspective* (London, 1990).

Malcolmson, R. and S. Mastoris, *The English Pig – A History* (London, 1998).

Malik, Kenan, *Man, Beast and Zombie* (London, 2000).

Mason, I.L., *Evolution of Domesticated Animals* (London, 1984).

Matthews, S., Explanations for the Outbreak of Cattle Plague in Cheshire in 1865–1866: Fear of the Wrath of the Lord, *Northern History*, XLIII: March 2006, 117–134.

Massehaele, J., 'Transport Costs in Medieval England', *The Economic Historical Review*, New Series, Vol 46, No 2, May 1993, 266–279.

Menache, Sophia, 'Hunting and attachment to dogs in the Pre-Modern Period' in A.L. Podberscek, E.S. Paul and J.A. Serpell (eds) *Companion Animals and Us* (Cambridge, 2000), 42–60.

Mullet, C.F., 'The Cattle Distemper in Mid-Eighteenth-Century England', *Agricultural History*, Vol. 20, No. 3 (Jul., 1946), pp. 144–165.

——, 'Public Baths and Health in England, Sixteenth to Eighteenth Century', *Supplement to the Bulletin of the History of Medicine* (Baltimore, 1946), p. 24.

——, 'Gervase Markham: Scientific Amateur', *ISIS*, Vol. 35, No 2 (Spring 1944) 106–118.

Mullin, M.H., Mirrors and Windows: Sociocultural Studies of Human-Animal Relationships, *Annual Review of Anthropology*, Vol 28, (1999), 201–224.

Murdy, W.H., Anthropocentrism: A Modern Version', *Science*, March, 1975, Vol 187, 1168–1172.

Naumova, E.N. 'Mystery of Seasonality: Getting the Rhythm of Nature', *Journal of Public Health Policy* (2006), 27, 2–12.

Nettleton, Sarah, *The Sociology of Health and Illness* (Cambridge, 1996).

Nutton, Vivian, *Ancient Medicine* (London, 2004).

O'Gorman, Frank, *The Long Eighteenth Century: British Political & Social History 1688–1832* (London, 2005).

Overton, Mark, *Agricultural Revolution in England: The transformation of the agrarian economy 1500–1850* (Cambridge, 1996).

——, The Diffusion of Agricultural Innovations in Early Modern England: Turnips and Clover in Norfolk and Suffolk, 1580-1740, *Transactions of the Institute of British Geographers*, New Series, Vol. 10, No. 2 (1985), pp 205–221.

Pattison, I., *The British Veterinary Profession 1791–1948* (London, 1984).

Pearson, D., *Provenance Research in Book History: A Handbook* (London, 1994).

Pollington, S. *Leechcraft: Early English Charms, Plantlore and Healing* (Trowbridge, 2000).

Porter, Dorothy and Roy Porter, *Patients Progess: Doctors and Doctoring in Eighteenth-Century England* (Oxford, 1989).

Porter, Roy, 'Civilisation and Disease: Medical Ideology in the Enlightenment' in J. Black and J. Gregory (eds) *Culture, Politics and Society in Britain 1660–1800* (Manchester, 1991).

——, 'Cleaning up the Great Wen: Public Health in Eighteenth Century London', *Medical History*, Supplement No. 11, 1991: 61–75.

——, *Health for Sale: Quackery in England 1660–1850* (Manchester, 1989).

——, 'The Patient in England, c.1660–c.1800' in Andrew Wear (ed.) *Medicine in Society* (Cambridge, 1992), 91–118.

——, 'Man, Animals and Medicine at the Time of the Founding of the Royal Veterinary College' in A.R. Mitchell (ed.) *History of the Healing Professions*, 3 (London, 1993), 19–30.

——, *The Greatest Benefit to Mankind: A Medical History of Humanity from Antiquity to the Present* (London, 1997).

Post, J.D., 'Climactic Variability and the European Morality Wave of the Early 1740's', *Journal of Interdisciplinary History*, XV (Summer, 1984), pp. 2–9.

Prince, Leslie B., *The Farrier and His Craft. The History of the Worshipful Company of Farriers* (London, 1980).

Pugh, Leslie P., *From Farriery to Veterinary Medicine 1785–1795* (Cambridge, 1962).

——, 'From Farriery to Veterinary Medicine', *Veterinary History*, 4 (1974–75), 10–16.

Raber, K. 'Nation and Race in Horsemanship Treatises' in K. Raber and T.J. Tucker (eds) *The Culture of the Horse: Status, Discipline and Identity in the Early Modern World* (Basingstoke, 2005), 225–243.

Rawcliffe, Carole, *Medicine and Society in Later Medieval England* (Stroud, 1995).

Reay, Barry, *Popular Cultures in England 1550–1750* (London, 1998).

Riedel, S. S. Riedel, 'Edward Jenner and the history of smallpox and vaccination', *Proceedings* (2005 January); 18(1): 21–25.

Ritvo, Harriet, *The Animal Estate* (Cambridge, MA, 1987).

Robyns, R., 'Medieval Astrology and the Buke of the Sevyne Sagis', *Forum for Modern Language Studies*, 38, No 4 (October 2002), 420–434.

Room, A. *The Naming of Animals: an appellative reference to domestic, work and show animals real and fictional* (London, 1993).

Ruckebusch, Y., 'A Historical Profile of Veterinary Pharmacology and Therapeutics', *Historia Medicinae Veterinariae*, 20 (1995), 49–80.

Ryder, M.L. *Sheep and Man* (London, 1983).

Salisbury, Joyce E., *The Beast Within: Animals in the Middle Ages* (London, 1994).

Schwabe, Calvin W., *Veterinary Medicine and Human Health* (Baltimore, 1984).

Serpell J., *In the Company of Animals: A study of human-animal relationships* (Cambridge, 1996).

Sharpe, Kevin, *Reading Revolutions: The Politics of Reading in Early Modern England* (New Haven, Conn., 2000).

Sigerist, H. *A History of Medicine*, I (Oxford, 1951).

Siraisi, Nancy, *Medieval & Early Renaissance Medicine* (Chicago, 1990).

Simonton, Deborah, *A History of European Women's Work 1700 to the Present* (London, 1998), p. 20 and H. Barker, 'Women and Work' in H. Barker and E. Chalus (eds) *Women's History, 1700–1850* (Abingdon, 2005).

Slack, Paul, 'Mirrors of Health and Treasures of Poor Men: The Uses of the Vernacular Medical Literature of Tudor England' in Charles Webster (ed.) *Health, Medicine and Mortality in the Sixteenth Century*, (Cambridge, 1979), 237–74.

Smith, Sir Frederick, *The Early History of Veterinary Literature and its British Development*, Vol. I (London, 1919).

——, *The Early History of Veterinary Literature*, Vol. II (London, 1924).

Smithcors, F.J., The History of Some Current Problems in Animal Disease: III. Rinderpest *Veterinary Medicine*, Vol LI, No 6 (June 1956), 249–56.

——, *Evolution of the Veterinary Art: A Narrative Account to 1850* (London, 1958).

——, *The American Veterinary Profession* (Ames, 1963).

——, 'Some Early Veterinary Therapies', *Veterinary Heritage*, 18 (1995), 48–52.

Soulsby, E.J.L., *Royal Society of Medicine News*, 15 September 1998.

Spinage, C.A., *Cattle Plague: A History* (New York, 2003).

Spufford, Margaret, *Small Books and Pleasant Histories: Popular Fiction and its Readership in Seventeenth-Century England* (Cambridge, 1981).

——, 'First Steps in Literacy: The Reading and Writing Experiences of the Humblest Seventeenth-Century Autobiographers', *Social History*, 4, 3 (1979), pp 407–35.

——, *Contrasting Communities: English Villagers in the Sixteenth and Seventeenth Centuries* (Cambridge, 1974).

Stapleton, B, 'Inherited Poverty and Life-Cycle Poverty: Odiham, Hampshire, 1650–1850', *Social History*, Vol. 18, No. 3 (Oct., 1993), pp. 339–355.

Swabe, Joanna, 'The Burden of Beasts: A Historical Sociological Study of Changing Human-Animal Relations and the Rise of the Veterinary Regime (Amsterdam, 1997).

Teigen, P.M., 'Reading and Writing Veterinary History', Veterinary Heritage, 24, no., 1 (May 2001).

Thagard, P., 'Why Astrology is a Pseudoscience', The Philosophy of Science Association, I (1978), pp. 233–4.

Thulesius, O., Nicholas Culpeper: English Physician and Astrologer (London, 1992).

Thirsk, Joan (ed.), The Agrarian History of England and Wales: Vol.II, (Cambridge, 1985).

Thomas, Keith, Man and the Natural World: Changing Attitudes in England 1500–1800 (London, 1983).

——, Religion and the Decline of Magic (London, 1991).

Torrey, E.F. and R.H.Yolken Beasts of the Earth: Animals, Humans and Disease (London, 2005).

Toussaint-Samat, M. History of Food, (trans.) A. Bell (New York, 1992).

Turner, B.S., The Government of the Body: Medical Regimens and the Rationalization of the Body' The British Journal of Sociology, Vol 33, No 2 (June 1982), 254–269.

Underdown, David, 'Regional Cultures? Local Variations in Popular Culture in the Early Modern Period' in T. Harris (ed.) Popular Culture in England, c.1500–1850 (London, 1995), pp. 28–48.

Voigts, L.E., 'Scientific and Medical Books' in J. Griffiths and D.A. Pearsall (eds.) Book production and publishing in Britain 1375–1475 (Cambridge, 1989), pp. 345–402.

Voigts, L.E. and M.R. McVaugh, 'A Latin Technical Phlebotomy and Its Middle English Translation', Transactions of the American Philosophical Society, New Ser., Vol. 74, 2 (1984) 1–69.

Walsham, Alexandra, Providence in Early Modern England (Oxford, 2001).

Wear, Andrew, Religious Beliefs and Medicine in Early Modern England' in H. Marland and M. Pelling (eds.) The Task of Healing: Medicine, Religion and Gender in England and the Netherlands 1450-1800 (Rotterdam, 1996).

——, Knowledge & Practice in English Medicine, 1550–1680 (Cambridge, 2000).

Webster, Charles, The Great Instauration: Science, Medicine and Reform 1626–1660 (New York, 1976).

Wendt, L.M., Dogs: A Historical Journey (New York, 1996).

White, Kevin, An Introduction to the Sociology of Health and Illness (London, 2007).

Wilkinson, Lise, Animals and Disease: An Introduction to the History of Comparative Medicine (Cambridge, 1992).

——, Rinderpest and Mainstream Infectious Disease Concepts in the Eighteenth Century, Medical History, (April 1984), 28(2), 129–250.

Wilson, D.,'Animal Ideas', Proceedings of the American Philosophy Association, Vol 69, 2, (November 1995), 7–25.

Wrightson, Keith, Earthly Necessities: Economic Lives in Early Modern Britain 1450–1750 (London, 2002).

INDEX

History of Science
and Medicine Library

ISSN 1872-0684

1. FRUTON, J.S. *Fermentation. Vital or Chemical Process?* 2006.
   ISBN 978 90 04 15268 7
2. PIETIKAINEN, P. *Neurosis and Modernity.* The Age of Nervousness in Sweden,
   2007. ISBN 978 90 04 16075 0
3. ROOS, A. *The Salt of the Earth.* Natural Philosophy, Medicine, and Chymistry in
   England, 1650-1750. 2007. ISBN 978 90 04 16176 4
4. EASTWOOD, B.S. *Ordering the Heavens.* Roman Astronomy and Cosmology in
   the Carolingian Renaissance. 2007. ISBN 978 90 04 16186 3 (Published as
   Vol. 8 in the subseries *Medieval and Early Modern Science*)
5. LEU, U.B., R. KELLER & S. WEIDMANN. *Conrad Gessner's Private Library.* 2008.
   ISBN 978 90 04 16723 0
6. HOGENHUIS, L.A.H. *Cognition and Recognition: On the Origin of Movement.*
   Rademaker (1887-1957): A Biography. 2009. ISBN 978 90 04 16836 7
7. DAVIDS, C.A. *The Rise and Decline of Dutch Technological Leadership.* Technology,
   Economy and Culture in the Netherlands, 1350-1800 (2 vols.). 2008.
   ISBN 978 90 04 16865 7 (Published as Vol. 1 in the subseries *Knowledge Infra-
   structure and Knowledge Economy*)
8. GRELLARD, C. & A. ROBERT (EDS.). *Atomism in Late Medieval Philosophy and
   Theology.* 2009. ISBN 978 90 04 17217 3 (Published as Vol. 9 in the subseries
   Medieval and Early Modern Science)
9. FURDELL, E.L. *Fatal Thirst.* Diabetes in Britain until Insulin. 2009.
   ISBN 978 90 04 17250 0
10. STRANO, G., S. JOHNSTON, M. MINIATI & A. MORRISON-LOW (EDS.). *European
    Collections of Scientific Instruments, 1550-1750.* 2009. ISBN 978 90 04 17270 8
    (Published as Vol. 1 in the subseries *Scientific Instruments and Collections*)
11. NOWACKI, H. & W. LEFÈVRE (EDS.). *Creating Shapes in Civil and Naval Architec-
    ture.* A Cross-Disciplinary Comparison. 2009. ISBN 978 90 04 17345 3
12. CHABÁS, J. & B.R. GOLDSTEIN (EDS.). *The Astronomical Tables of Giovanni
    Bianchini.* 2009. ISBN 978 90 04 17615 7 (Published as Vol. 10 in the subseries
    Medieval and Early Modern Science)
13. EAGLETON, C. *Monks, Manuscripts and Sundials: The Navicula in Medieval
    England.* 2010. ISBN 978 90 04 17665 2
14. HILL CURTH, L. *The Care of Brute Beasts.* A Social and Cultural Study of Veteri-
    nary Medicine in Early Modern England. 2010. ISBN 978 90 04 17995 0
15. GODDU, A. *Copernicus and the Aristotelian Tradition.* Education, Reading, and
    Philosophy in Copernicus's Path to Heliocentrism. 2010.
    ISBN 978 90 04 18107 6